Table of Contents

Preface

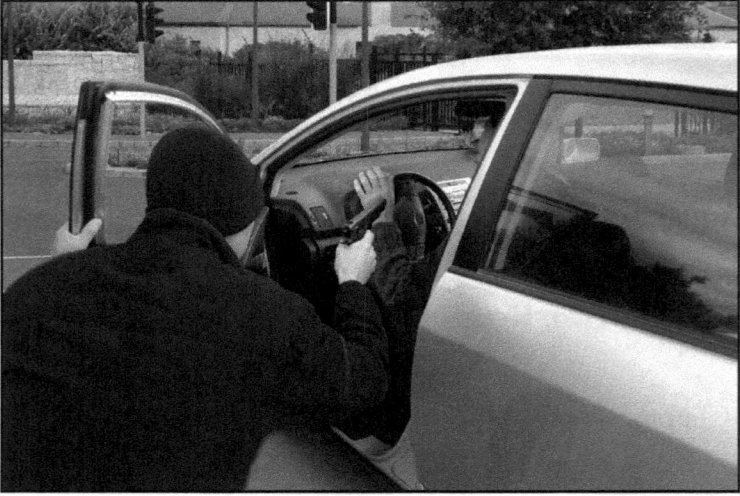

For most people, the mere though of self-defense conjures up images of law abiding citizens learning the physical skills necessary to defend themselves against a criminal assault. However, the truth is, real self-defense is a state of mind. A way of thinking and a way of living your life!

Self-Defense Tips and Tricks takes you inside the criminal's mind and arms you with his tactics and techniques allowing you to beat him at his own game by stopping him dead in his tracks.

The goal of this book is to make you acutely aware of the many hidden dangers that exist on the streets, in your homes, and at the workplace. It's not intended to frighten you or make you paranoid. But rather, educate you with the knowledge, skills and attitude necessary to protect yourself and your family against all forms of violent crime.

The self-defense tips and solutions featured in this book can be used by men and women of all ages. Some readers might find some of the suggestions in this book a bit unusual or unconventional. This is understandable and expected. However, the important point is for you to adopt what works for you and reject the ones that don't fit into your lifestyle. The late Bruce Lee put it best when he said, "absorb what is useful, reject what is useless, add what is specifically your own."

You will also discover that a good portion of this book focuses on avoidance skills and techniques. After all, the highest form of self-defense is avoiding danger altogether.

However, for those of you who are looking for a more robust self-defense solution, I strongly encourage you to read my other book, *When Seconds Count: Self-Defense for the Real World.*

Stay Safe!

- Sammy Franco

Important!

Some of the information and techniques presented in this book can be dangerous and could lead to serious injury. The author, publisher, and distributors of this book disclaim any liability from loss, injury, or damage, personal or otherwise, resulting from the information and procedures in this book. This book is for academic study only.

It is the reader's responsibility to research and comply with all local, state and federal laws.

SELF DEFENSE
Tips & Tricks

Practical Self-Defense Solutions for the Street, Home, Workplace and Travel

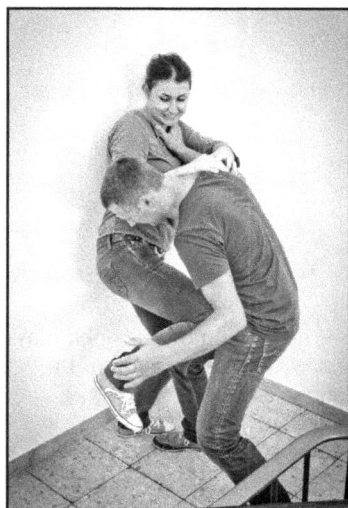

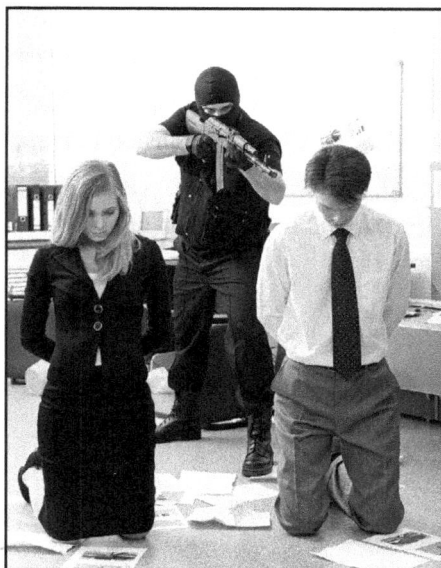

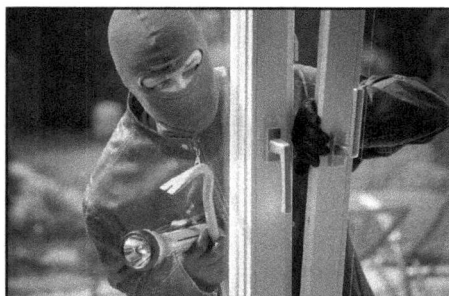

SAMMY FRANCO

Self-Defense Tips and Tricks

Also by Sammy Franco

Maximum Damage: Hidden Secrets Behind brutal Fighting Combinations
Kubotan Power
The Complete Body Opponent Bag Book
Heavy Bag Training: Boxing, Mixed Martial Arts & Self-Defense
Gun Safety: For Home Defense and Concealed Carry
Out of the Cage: A Complete Guide to Beating a Mixed Martial Artist on the Street
Warrior Wisdom: Inspiring Ideas from the World's Greatest Warriors
Judge, Jury and Executioner
Savage Street Fighting: Tactical Savagery as a Last Resort
Feral Fighting
War Craft: Street Fighting Tactics of the War Machine
War Machine: How to Transform Yourself Into a Vicious and Deadly Street Fighter
The Bigger They Are, The Harder They Fall
First Strike: End a Fight in Ten Seconds or Less
1001 Street Fighting Secrets
When Seconds Count: Self-Defense for the Real World
Killer Instinct: Unarmed Combat for Street Survival
Street Lethal: Unarmed Urban Combat

Self-Defense Tips and Tricks
Copyright © 2014 by Sammy Franco
ISBN 978-0-9890382-8-7
Printed in the United States of America

Published by Contemporary Fighting Arts, LLC.
P.O. Box 84028
Gaithersburg, Maryland 20883 USA
Phone: (301) 279-2244
Visit us Online at: www.sammyfranco.com

For author interviews or publicity information, please send inquiries in care of the publisher.

Chapter One
Street Smart Safety

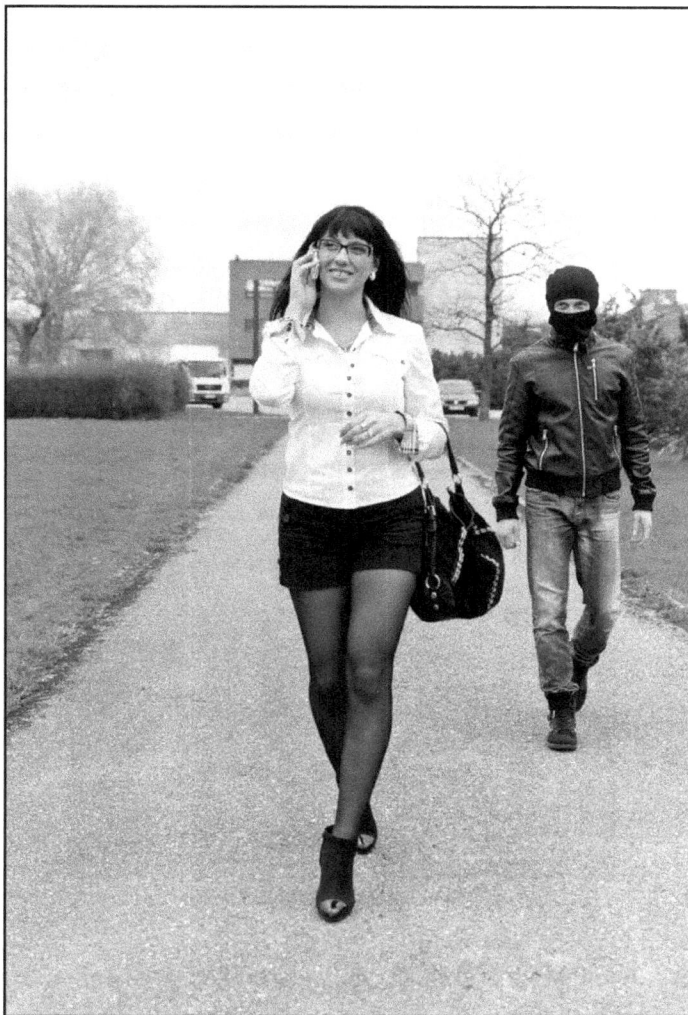

Self-Defense Tips and Tricks

- Never take your personal safety for granted.

- Be alert and aware of your surroundings at all times.

- Always turn wide corners. Do not go around corners within 5 feet of a wall, building, shrubbery, etc.

- Do not walk down the street looking lost, fatigued, uncertain, or preoccupied. Assertive body language is essential. Keep your head up and walk with confidence and purpose, even if you are lost.

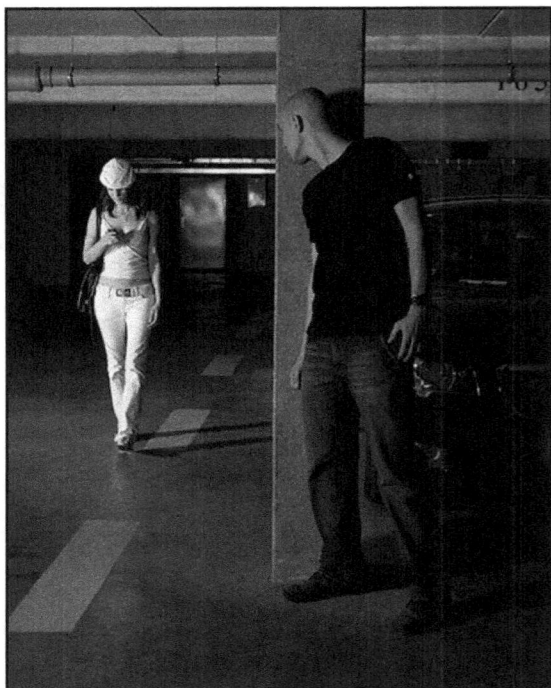

Do not walk down the street looking lost, fatigued, uncertain, or preoccupied.

- Assume that violence can, and very well may, occur anywhere.

- Constantly scan your environment, thoroughly and quickly noting potential problems.

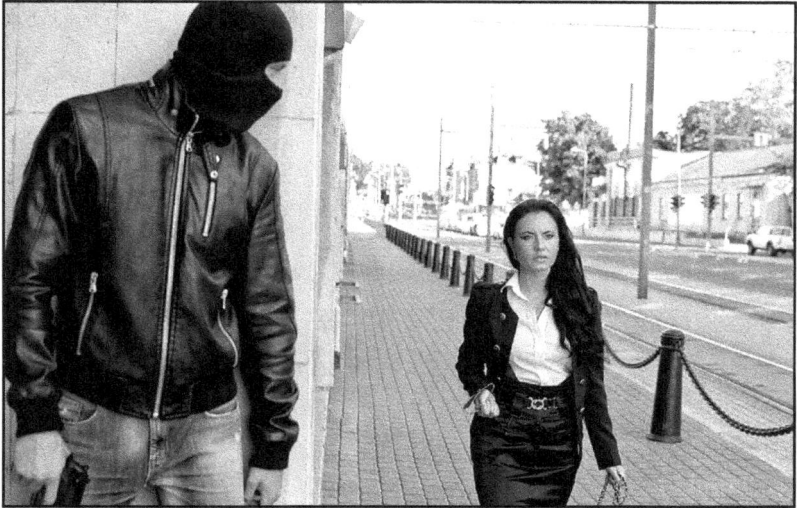

To improve your defensive reaction time against a possible attack, always turn wide corners. Do not go around corners within 5 feet of a wall or building.

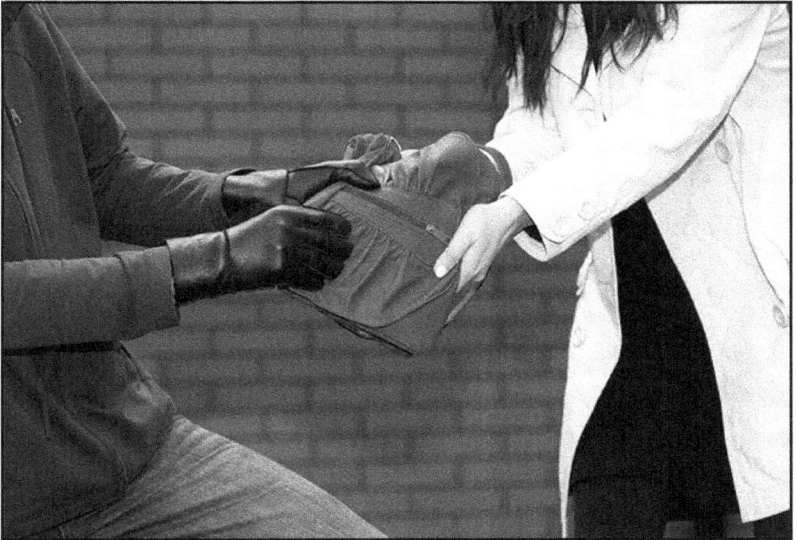

If you are confronted by a criminal forcibly demanding your possessions, give them up. Material items can always be replaced.

Self-Defense Tips and Tricks

• When walking in the streets, avoid high-crime areas.

• When entering a dark environment, allow a few seconds for your eyes to adjust before moving on.

• When walking down the street, if something doesn't feel right, listen to your instincts and get the heck out of there.

• Get into the habit of walking briskly.

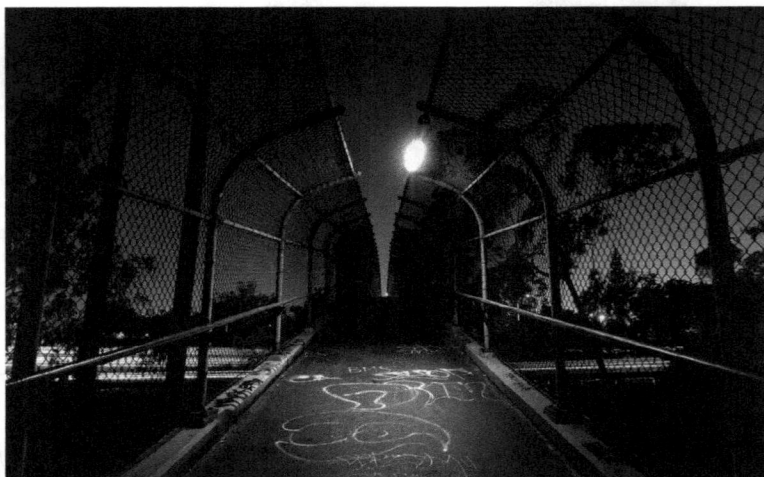

Stay in well-lit areas. However, if you must walk in a dark environment, allow a few seconds for your eyes to adjust before moving on.

• Familiarize yourself with ambush zones and avoid them whenever possible. Ambush zones are strategic locations (in everyday environments) from which an assailant can launch a surprise attack. Ambush zones can be found and exploited in unfamiliar and familiar environments, even in your home, and in unpopulated and populated areas. An ambush zone can be set in a dark or poorly lit area as well as in a well-lit location. Ambush zones can be established in a variety of common places: under, behind, or around trees, utility boxes and shrubs; under or around beds, corners, trash dumpsters, doorways, walls, tables, automobiles, trash cans, rooftops, bridges, ramps

4

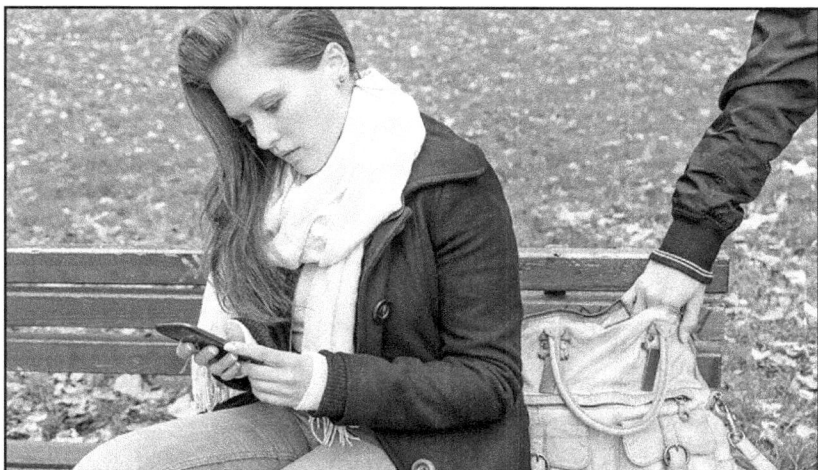

When in public places, stay alert at all times and don't let your cellphone distract you from your environment.

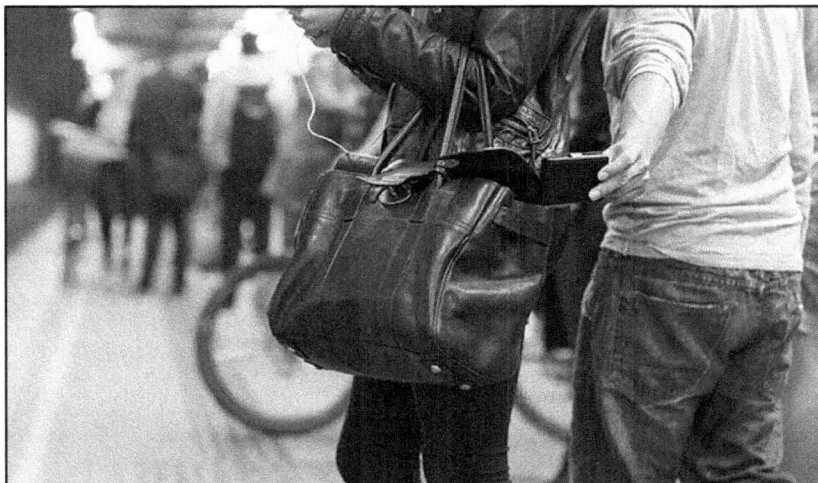

Listening to music on your phone can also distract you from criminal activity.

and mailboxes. Now is the time to familiarize yourself with these various types of ambush zones and avoid them whenever possible.

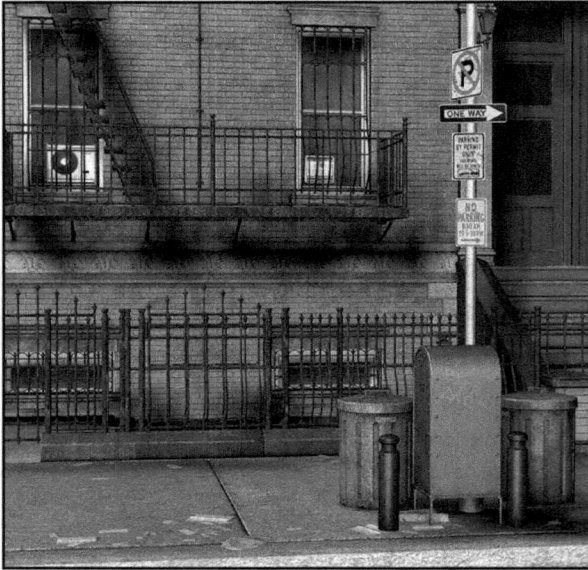

How many ambush zones do you see in this picture?

• If you think you are being followed when walking down a street, immediately cross the street at a 90-degree angle and observe the behavior of everyone else on the street. Remember, you can be followed or trailed from directions other that the one immediately behind you.

• If a car approaches you while you are walking down the street and you are harassed by the drivers, yell and run in the opposite direction.

• Never turn your back on a potential aggressor unless he is so far away he can't reach you before you get to safety.

• Don't argue with anyone, give offensive gestures, or engage in eye wars.

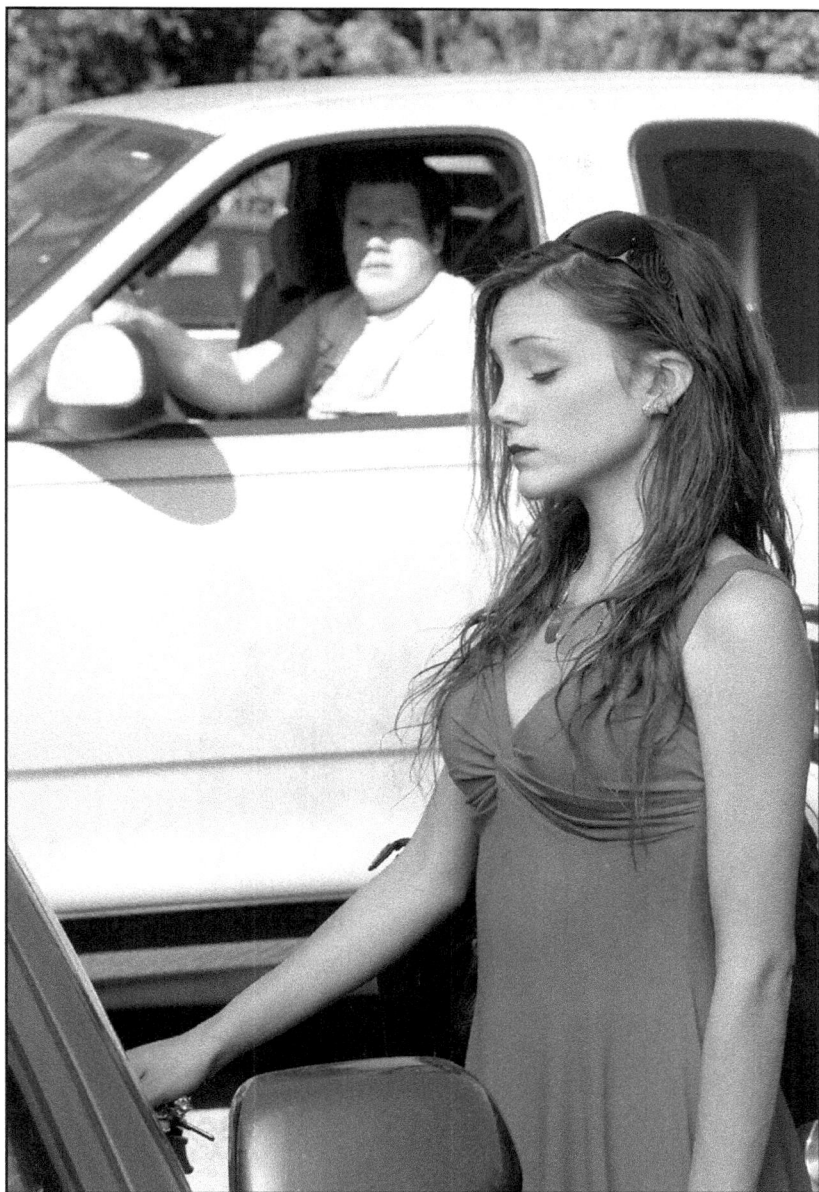

Assume the criminal predator is out there and he's watching you!

Self-Defense Tips and Tricks

• Don't display money or jewelry in public.

• Wear clothes and shoes that facilitate quick and free movement. Try to wear sneakers or shoes with low heels. If you are wearing high heels and are being chased, kick them off and run barefoot.

• Don't carry large amount of cash.

• Vary your travel routes. Constant patterns allow assailants to monitor your behavior, note the regularity of your schedule, and pick an opportune time for attack.

• Look strong and competent! Remember, criminals look for low risk targets.

• Learn to use store windows and other reflecting sources to note suspicious activity behind you.

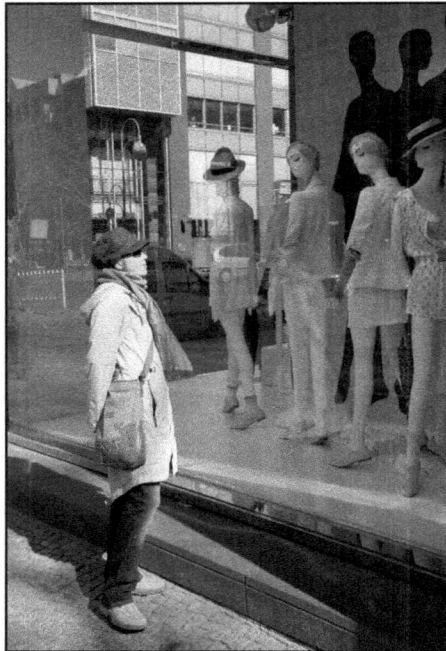

Learn to use store windows and other reflecting sources to note suspicious activity behind you.

• There is power in numbers, but don't be fooled into thinking that a group of people can't be victimized on the streets.

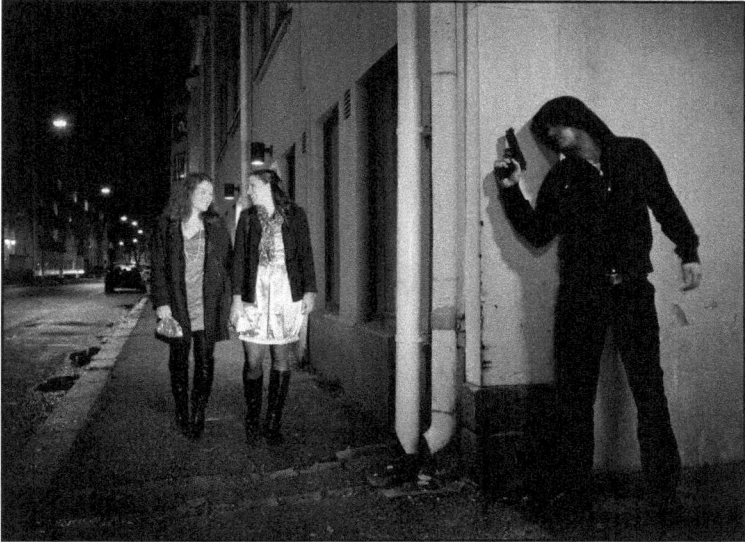

Don't be complacent just because you have a friend with you.

• If a physical confrontation with an assailant seems inevitable, then strike first, fast, repeatedly, and then escape.

• Do not be in denial about how dangerous and violent the streets can be.

• When visiting recreational facilities (beaches, parks, movie theaters, bars, etc.), avoid calling attention to yourself with loud or boisterous behavior.

• There is nothing cowardly about running away from danger. Escape or tactical retreat means to flee from the threat or danger safely and rapidly. For example, if you are being held hostage and your captor is distracted long enough for you to escape safely, then do it.

• Don't sleep on public transportation and try not to use it if fatigued or intoxicated.

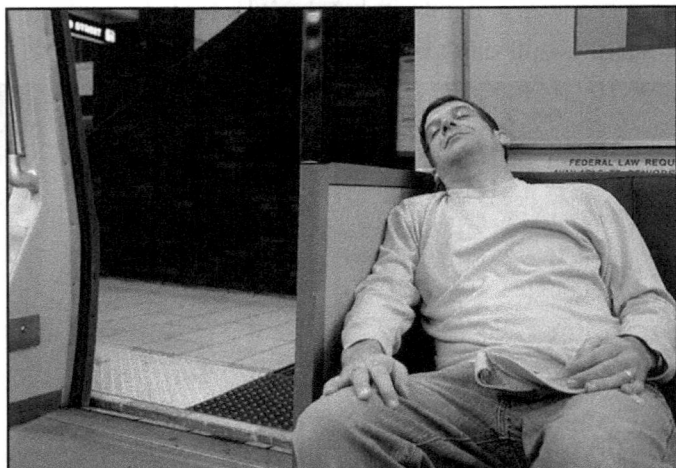

Avoid the tendency to doze off when traveling on the subway.

• Know your bus schedule to avoid long waits at the bus stop.

• When traveling on the subway, stay alert at all times.

• When exiting a bus, watch who is getting off with you and who is waiting at the stop.

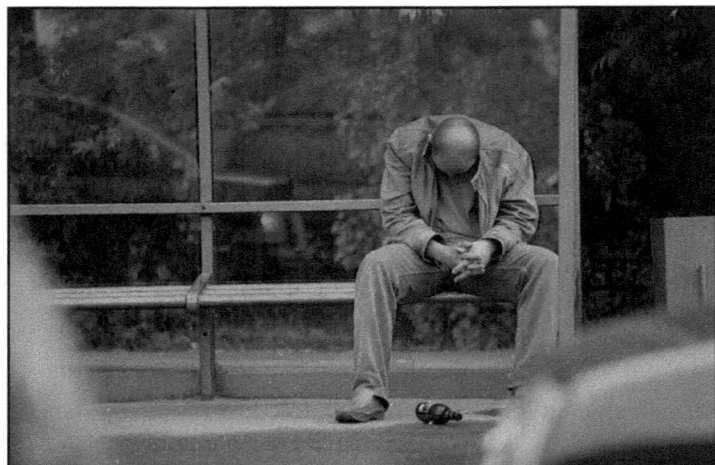

Always anticipate trouble. For example, see who is waiting at the bus stop before you get off of the bus.

• Walk, run, or jog in the opposite direction of traffic.

• Avoid tunnel vision when exercising or doing anything for that matter. Stay aware and alert.

• Avoid walking, biking, or jogging alone. Try to get a friend or family member to go with you.

• Plan your biking, jogging, and walking routes. Do not travel through dangerous areas containing a high number of high-risk ambush zones. If possible, let someone know what your route will be and how long you plan to be gone.

• If you must run or exercise outdoors in the evening, wear reflective clothing and don't wear earphones.

• If you must workout outdoors, such as jogging or bicycling, try to vary your route and avoid isolated areas.

• When running or jogging outdoors, try to avoid looking tired or exhausted from the workout. Look refreshed and energetic.

• Avoid running or jogging alone in the woods.

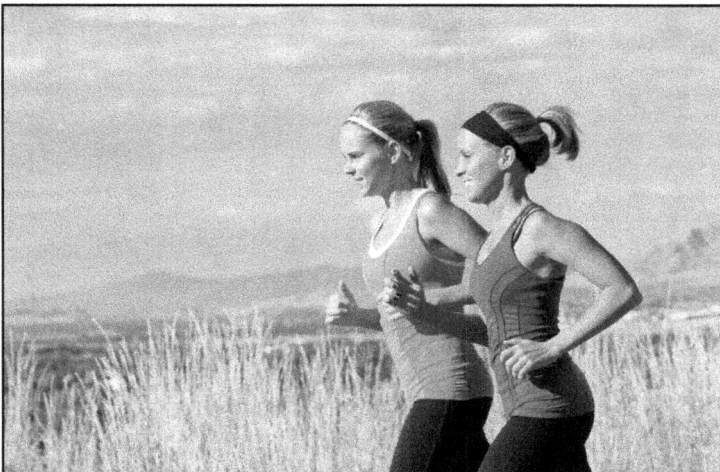

If possible, try to avoid working out alone. Try to get a friend or family member to go with you.

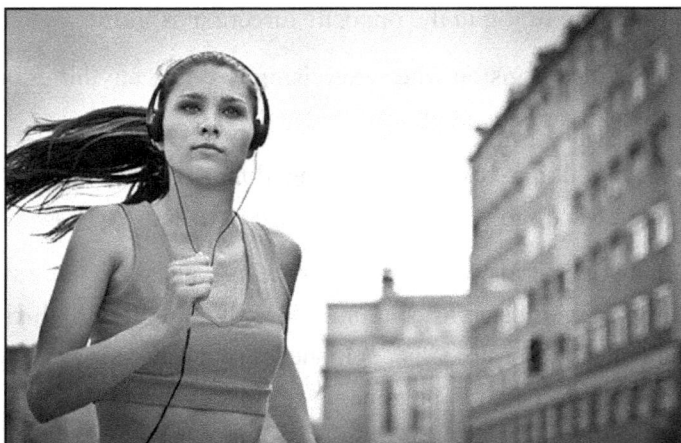

When working out outdoors, you must be able to see and hear everything that is going on around you. Leave the earphones at home.

• When training outdoors, always carry some form of identification with you. RoadID.com makes several great products for runners.

• When entering a taxi, observe the driver's identification card and make sure it matches his face. If there isn't a picture ID card, get out immediately.

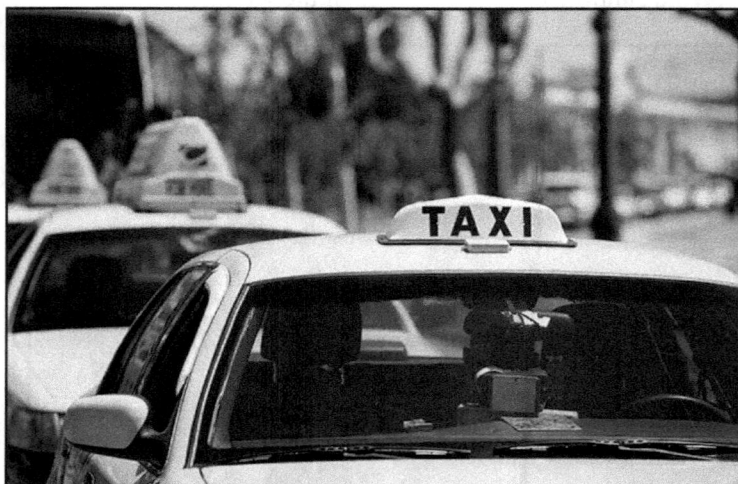

When entering a taxi, observe the driver's identification card and make sure it matches his face. If there isn't a picture ID card, get out immediately.

• If ever you feel uneasy in a taxi ask the driver to stop in a busy and familiar area, and get out immediately.

• Do not take shortcuts through alleys, parking lots, tunnels, parks, construction sites, or abandoned buildings.

• Be wary in public rest rooms.

• Do not carry more credit cards than you plan to use.

• Try to sit with your back to the wall in public places.

• When waiting for the elevator, stand approximately 6 feet away from the doors.

• Do not get on an elevator with a lone male stranger if you can avoid it. If you are about to exit an elevator and there is a suspicious person on the landing, do not exit the elevator. If you enter an elevator alone and a suspicious person joins you, get off immediately. If that's not possible, push a number of buttons for stops including the immediately available floor. If you are attacked on the elevator, push all the buttons. This will deny your attacker privacy.

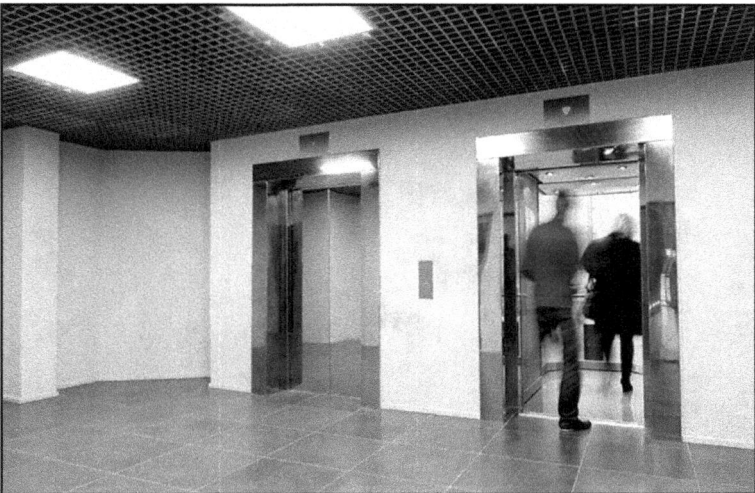

If possible, avoid getting on an elevator with a lone male stranger.

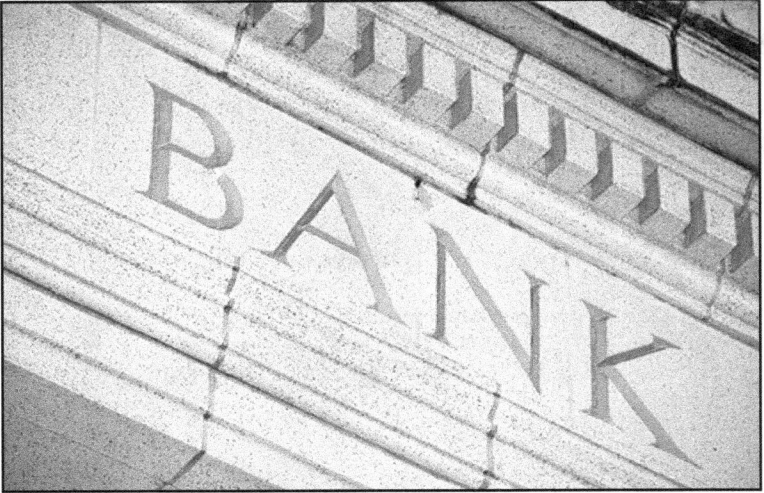

Banks are not safe havens. Make it a habit to always take a quick look inside before entering.

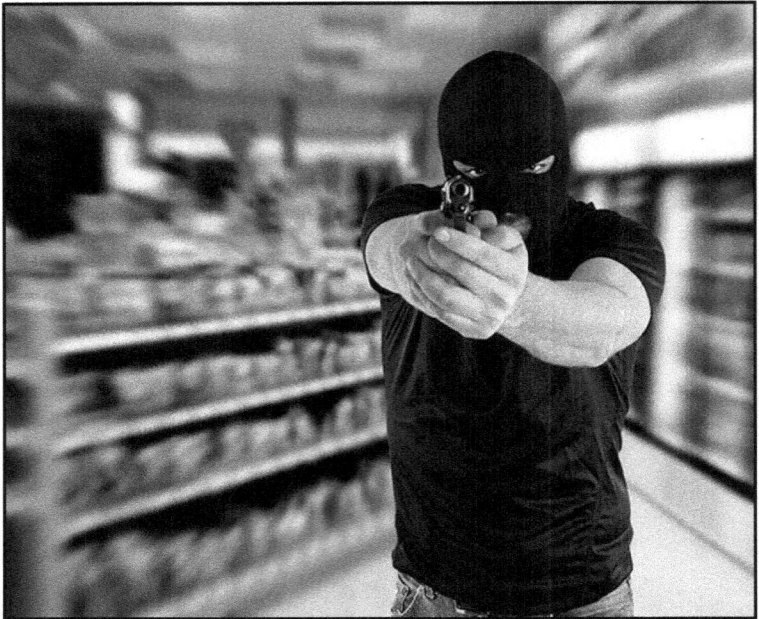

Be especially alert when entering convenient stores.

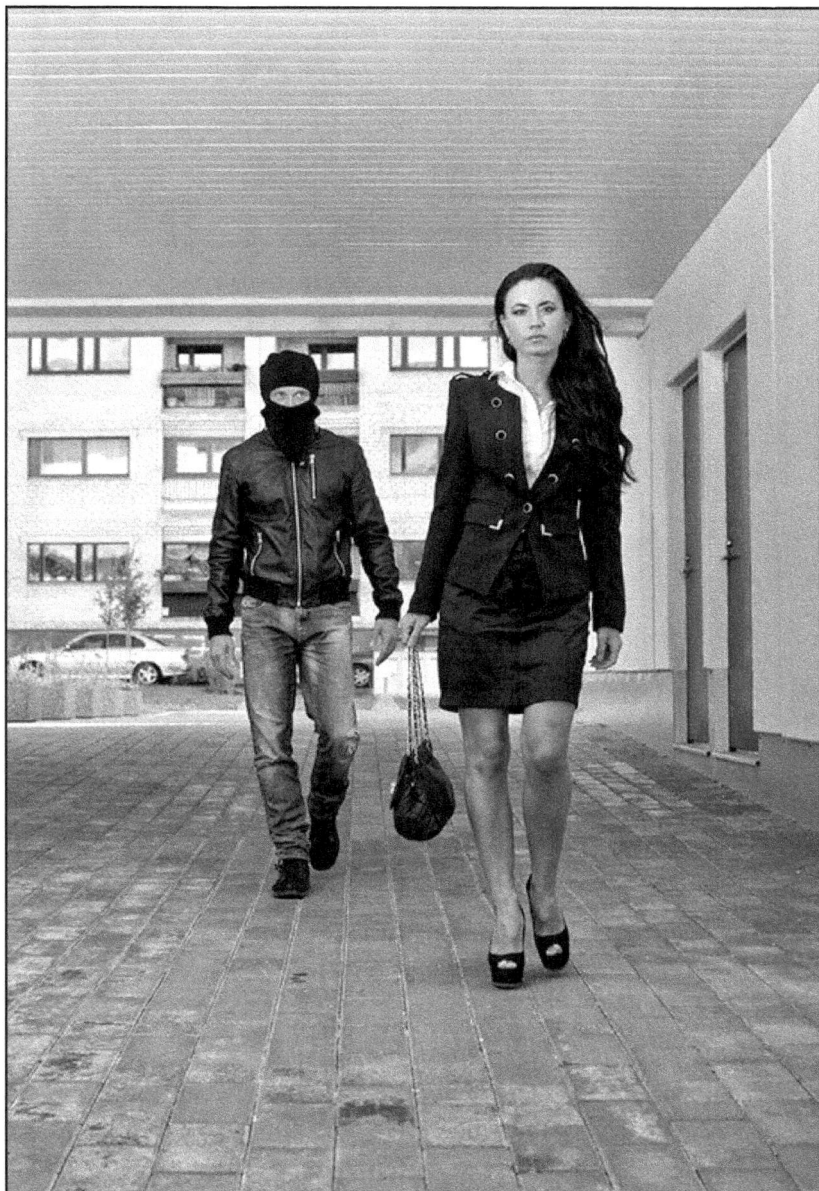

When walking on public streets, you want to avoid doing this! Remember, keep your purse close to your body with a firm grip and with the flap facing you.

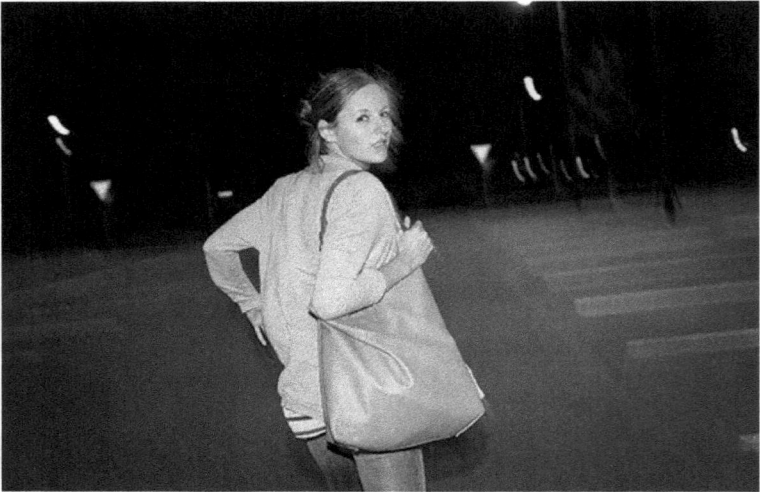

Get into the habit of looking over your shoulder, especially at night.

• Before entering convenience stores and banks, take a quick look inside to make sure no trouble is going down.

• When walking on public streets, keep your purse close to your body with a firm grip and with the flap facing you.

• Do not carry chemical sprays, stun guns, knives, or guns unless you have been trained adequately in their use.

• To avoid looking defenseless to a criminal, avoid overloading yourself with grocery bags and packages. If a stranger offers to help you, quickly and politely decline the offer.

• Know the escapes routes in familiar buildings. In unfamiliar

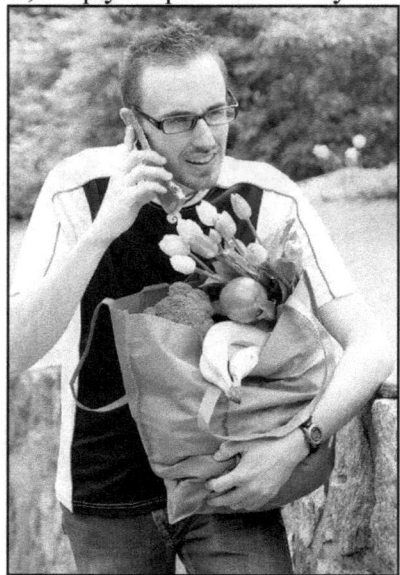

Avoid multi-tasking in public places. This is a criminal's dream come true.

buildings, look around for fire exits, kitchen routes, etc.

• If you are ever confronted with an exhibitionist flasher, don't react. This is what he wants. Just contact the police immediately.

• Destroy all credit card carbon copies before leaving an establishment.

• On public transportation sit in the aisle as close as possible to the driver. On subways, pick cars as close to the operator's car as possible.

• Try to stay in good shape. The quality of your life will improve and you will be better able to defend yourself.

• To avoid being pick pocketed, keep your wallet in your front pocket.

• If you must attend the movies alone, avoid sitting in the last few rows.

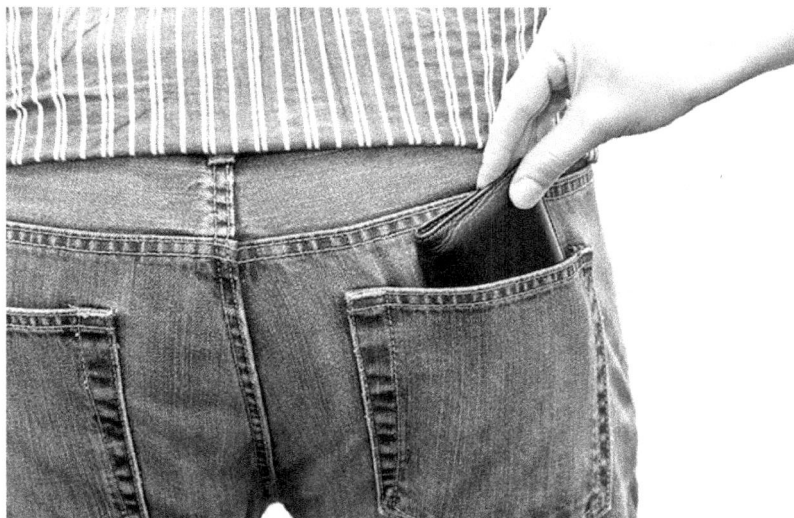

To avoid being pick pocketed, keep your wallet in your front pocket.

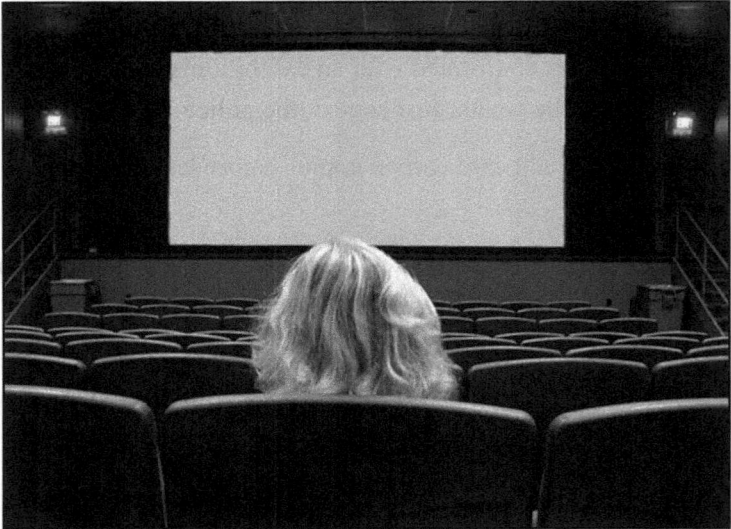

If you must attend the movies alone, avoid sitting in the last few rows.

• Never resist or fight for your possessions. Comply and hand it over. Stolen item can always be replaced.

• Try to avoid streets where groups of teenagers congregate.

• Never divulge personal information (name, age, home or work address, phone number) to any stranger.

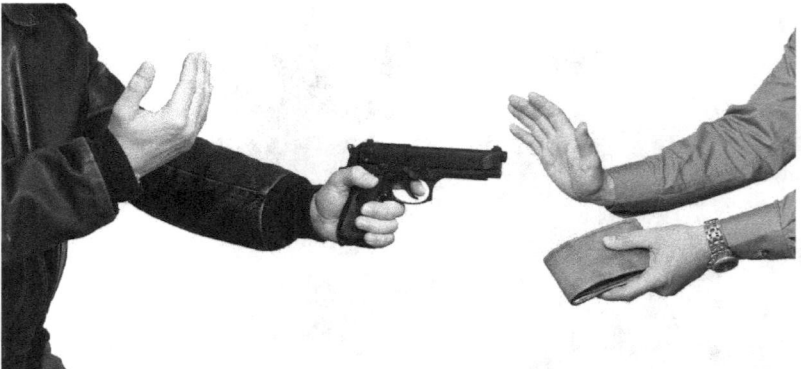

Comply means to obey the assailant's commands. For example, if you are held at gun point (out of disarming range) for the purpose of robbery, there is nothing to do but comply. Take out your wallet, take off your watch, hand over your car keys, do what you are told. Comply.

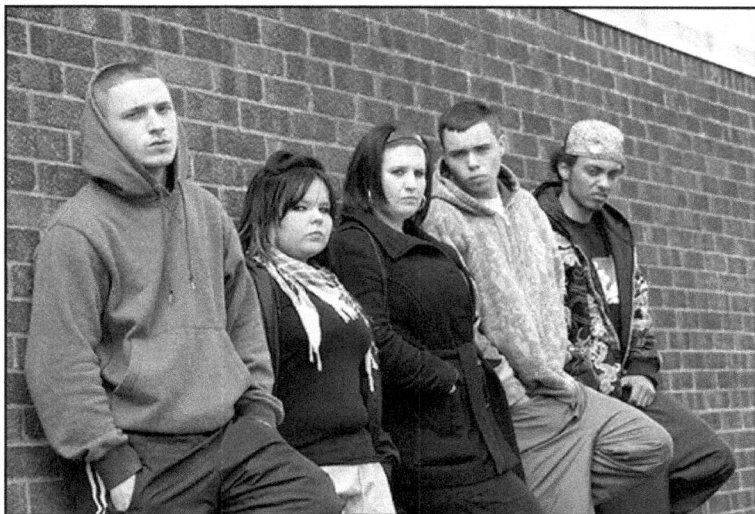

Never under estimate the destructive capability of a teenager.

• When walking the streets at night, try to travel in pairs or groups.

• If you are being attacked on the street, smash a store window to attract attention.

• Do not try to reason with a potential assailant unless you are buying time to escape, signaling for help, or setting up a counterattack.

• When making a purchase in a store, never recite your telephone number to the store cashier. Instead, write it down.

• It's a good idea to try and learn everything you can about your public transportation system. There might come a day when you may need to use it in an emergency.

• When going out, tell a family member, friend or roommate where you are going and when you are expected to return.

• When shopping, never leave your valuables unattended in a

19

fitting room. When grocery shopping, never leave your purse unattended in your cart.

• Avoid being kidnapped at all costs. If held at gunpoint, run in a serpentine pattern while screaming for help. The odds of being killed by a gunshot wound under these conditions are low.

• If you are kidnapped, remain as calm as possible. Don't argue, question, or lecture your captors. Wait for a solid opportunity to escape and take it. Don't hesitate, but don't attempt escape prematurely.

• If you are kidnapped prepare yourself for possible verbal and physical abuse, as well as lack of food, water, and sanitation.

• Consider carrying pepper spray or OC. Pepper spray, is an inflammatory agent that affects the assailants mucous membranes such as the eyes, nose, throat, and lungs. When OC is sprayed in a criminal space, it causes the eyes to swell shut, restricts breathing, and severely burned the mucous membranes. Vision is impaired for approximately 10 minutes, while breathing is restricted for about 30

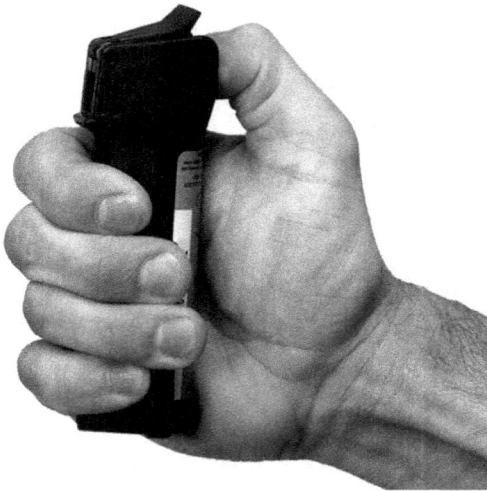

While pepper spray is very effective against criminals, remember that no single self-defense weapon will guarantee the safety of you or your family.

minutes. However, never carry pepper spray unless you are trained to use it.

• Don't be dependent on pepper spay. Aerosol canisters have also been known to clog and jam. Also, you cannot spray someone in a confined area like a car, bathroom stall, or small closet. Keep in mind that if the assailant holds his breath and closes his eyes, the spray won't stop him from attacking and injuring you. Above all, do not make the mistake of dependency. Remember, no single self-defense weapon will guarantee the safety of you and your family.

• Consider carrying personal safety weapons such as pepper spray, kubotans, stun guns, and even a whistle. Just be certain that you are trained to use them properly in a self-defense situation.

• Only use ATM machines in well-lighted, high-traffic areas. Never use a money machine in a remote area.

• When using a drive-thru ATM machine, keep a close eye on the side and rear view mirrors and always keep you car in gear with the foot on the break. If someone approaches you, drive off immediately.

• When getting money at machines or teller windows, put it away

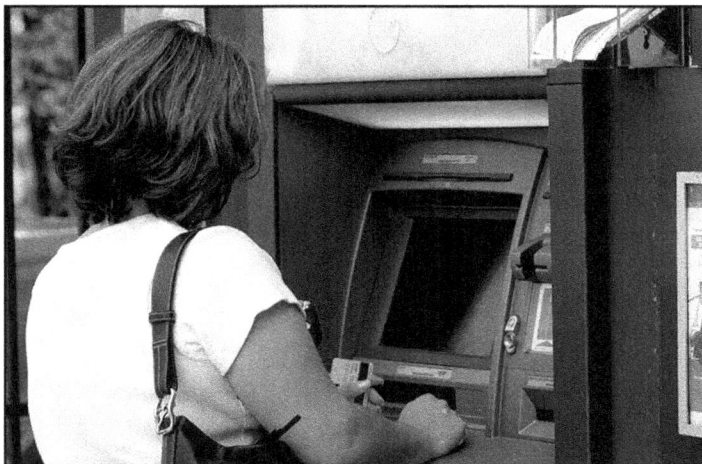

Be especially alert when using money machines.

before leaving.

• Don't allow strangers to stop you on the street.

• If you are being followed, always have a plan of action in mind. For example, you should know exactly where you need to go and what you would do if a dangerous situation occurs. If you live in the city, it is essential that you know where the nearest fire station or police station is located. Also, you should know how to contact the police or close friend in the event of an emergency. Finally, it's a good idea to know what businesses are open late so you could seek refuge if needed.

• If someone is following you, immediately let them know by turning around and looking at them. Let them know that you are suspicious and will not be taken by surprise.

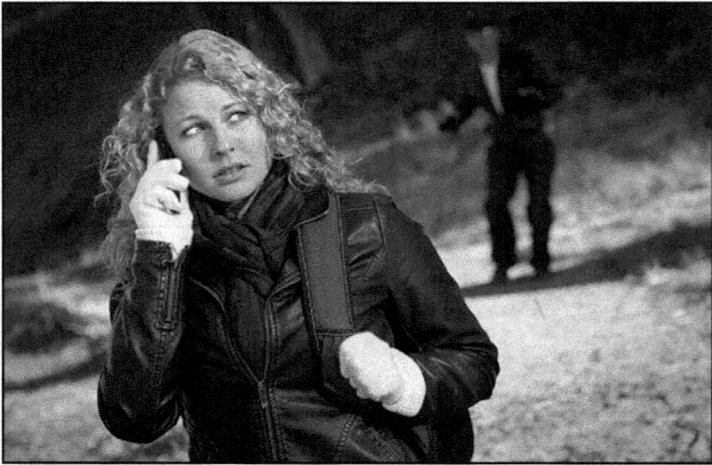

It's very important to have a plan of action in the event that you are being followed.

• Develop your sense of criminal awareness. Criminal awareness involves a general understanding and knowledge of the nature and dynamic of the criminal's motivations, mentalities, methods, and capabilities to perpetrate violent acts. By keeping yourself informed of global incidents through the media, official crime reports, and other sources, you will gain a necessary grasp of the types and trends of violent acts and the reasons behind them.

• How you dress in public is also important. If possible, try to avoid looking unique or glamorous. Your goal to simply blend in with everyone else. Avoid wearing bright colors and flashy jewelry or bling.

• Never drive into an unfamiliar neighborhood without a full tank of gas.

• If you witness a fight in the streets, call 911 and notify the police of the incident. If at all possible, try to avoid getting involved in the situation. Often in many cases, it's difficult to decipher who is a victim and who is the attacker.

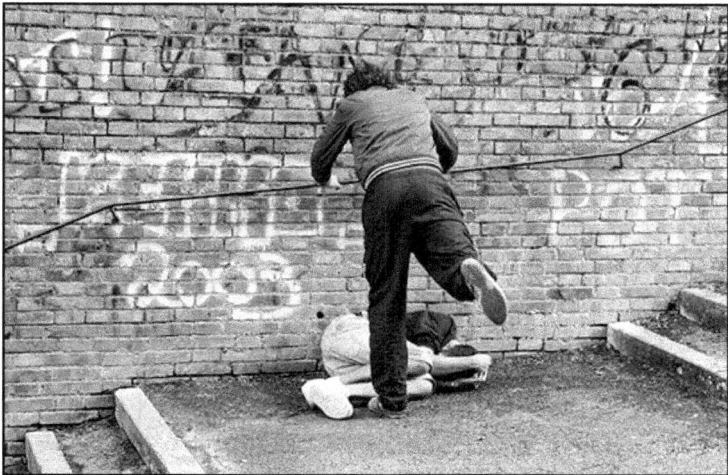

The decision to intervene in a street altercation is a personal one. Just remember, that many good Samaritans have died while trying to help others.

• If you ever have the opportunity, try to talk to police officers about their encounters with street criminals. Law enforcement people are generally very candid, and they can teach you a lot about the realities of street violence.

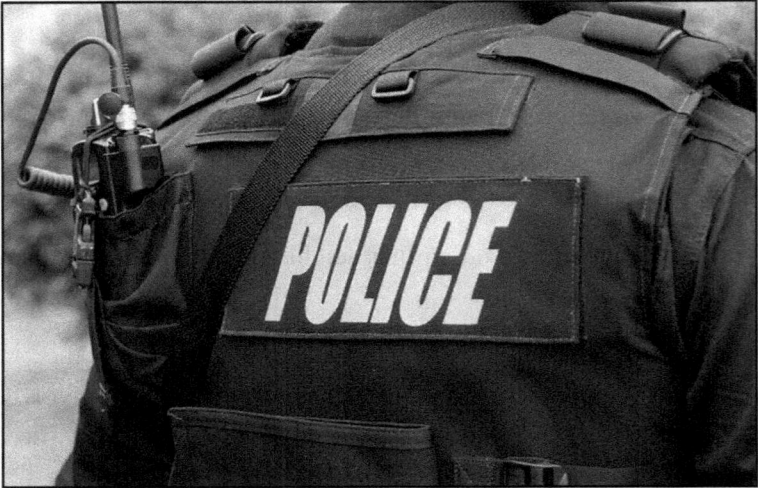

You would be amazed how much you can learn about violent crime by simply talking to the police.

• Self-awareness is a critical component of self-defense and personal protection. For example, it's important to know what aspects of your self provoke violence and which, if any would promote a proper reaction in a self-defense situation. For example, what are your physical strengths and weaknesses? Do you have any training in self-defense? Are you in shape? How do you handle stress? Do you panic or frighten easily? Are you likely to aggravate or diffuse a hostile situation? Are you passive or aggressive? Are you opinionated? Hot tempered? What is your age and gender? Does the nature of your occupation make you or your family vulnerable to different forms of criminal violence?

• When faced with a dangerous situation on the streets, the two most important factors to assess are the environment and the individual(s).

• Always know where the escape routes are in your immediate environment. Essentially, escape routes are various avenues or exits from a threatening situation. Some possible escape routes are windows, doors, fire escapes, gates, escalators, fences, walls, bridges, and staircases. But be careful that your version of an escape route doesn't lead you into a worse situation.

• Learn to identify barriers. A barrier is any object that obstructs the attackers path of attack. At the very least, barriers give you distance and some precious time, and they may give you some safety. The barrier must have a structural integrity to perform the particular function you assigned to it. Barriers may include such things as large desks, doors, automobiles, trash dumpsters, large trees, fences, walls, heavy machinery, and large vending machines. It really depends on the situation, but it's always a good idea to assess in advance any possible barriers when entering an unfamiliar environment.

• Learn how to use makeshift weapons. Makeshift weapons are common, everyday objects that can be converted into self-defense weapons. Like a barrier, makeshift weapons must be appropriate to the function of the signed it. Makeshift weapons include but are not

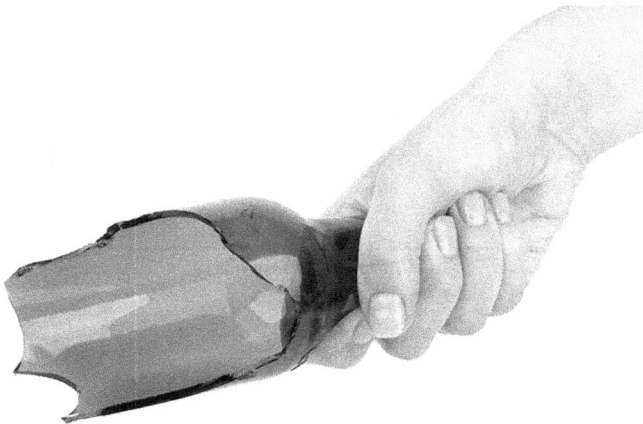

A broken beer bottle can be used as a makeshift weapon.

limited to: walking sticks, flashlights, bottles, hot liquids, briefcases, trashcan lids, screwdrivers, kitchen cutlery, scissors, ice scrapers, pens, etc.

• Your voice is a weapon. Yelling actually serves a strategic purpose in self-defense. Yelling while fighting back distracts, startles, and temporarily paralyzes your attacker. In some cases, it can cause them to freeze in his tracks, allowing you the split second advantage to deliver a debilitating strike.

• Every year read the uniform crime report or UCR. By keeping yourself informed through this official source, you will gain a necessary grasp of the types and trends of violence and crime. Pay particular attention to the demographic, seasonal, and regional variations in crime.

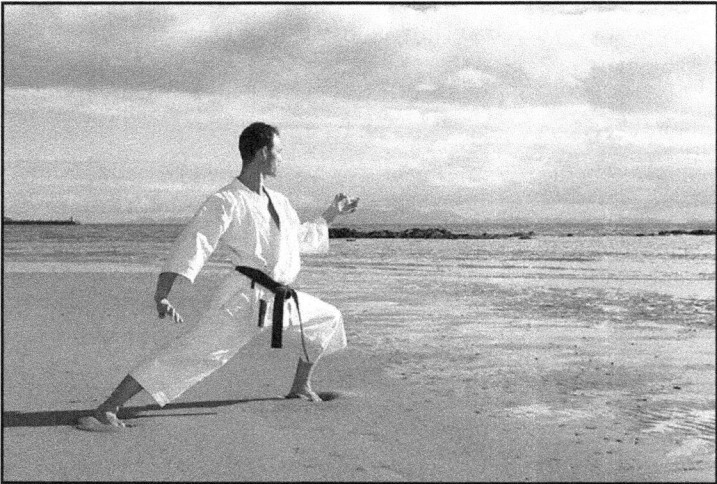

If you want to avoid potential problems, avoid practicing martial arts and self-defense in public places.

• If you study Karate, Kung-fu or mixed martial arts, avoid wearing your uniform or school t-shirt in public. Some people might interpret this as a dare or challenge to fight.

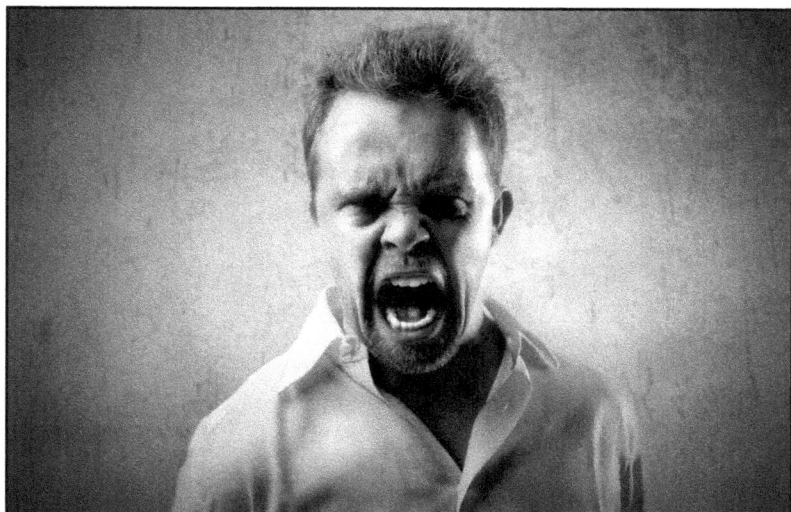

Many violent situations can be avoided by simply applying de-escalation skills.

• Learn how to de-escalate a hostile person. De-escalation is the strategic process of diffusing a potentially violent confrontation. The goal is to eliminate the possibility of an agitated individual resorting to physical violence. A self-defense instructor can teach you this.

• If you are involved in a violent assault, and once the confrontation is over and there is no apparent danger, conduct an immediate inventory of your body. Quickly scan your torso, hands, arms, legs, and feet for any signs of injury. Run your hands down your face and over your head and neck to check for blood. If the attack occurred at home, also check the other members of your household for any sign of injury. For those of you who might think it's silly and unnecessary to check yourself, think again. Many times people are seriously injured after a fight and don't even know it because the adrenaline rush from the flight-or flight response shuts off pain.

• If your attacker escaped from the scene, try to write down his or her description. Be sure to include their height, weight, clothing, weapon, car model, license tag number, or anything else that might

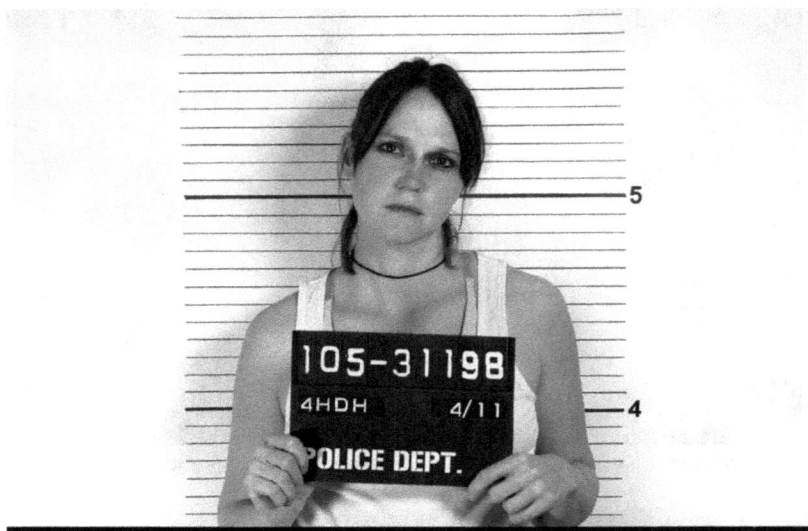

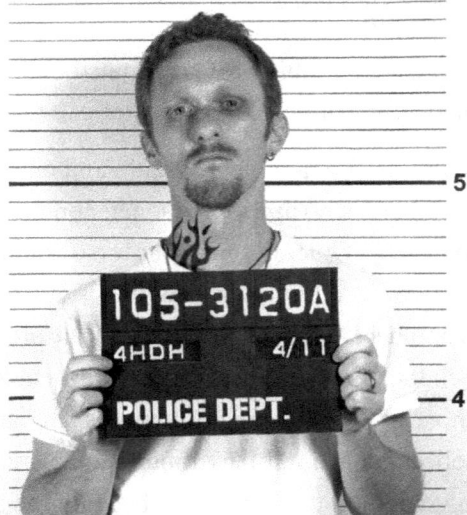

Jotting down information about your assault is important because the shock of a violent altercation usually makes victims forget many important details about the attacker and the crime itself.

assist the police in apprehending him. Jotting down this information is important because the shock of a violent altercation usually makes victims forget many important details about the attacker and the crime itself.

• Read the newspaper. Your local newspaper can provide you with a wealth of information about violence and crime. Get into the habit of reading it regularly. Pay close attention to what you are reading and find out the motivations, mentalities, and methods of street criminals.

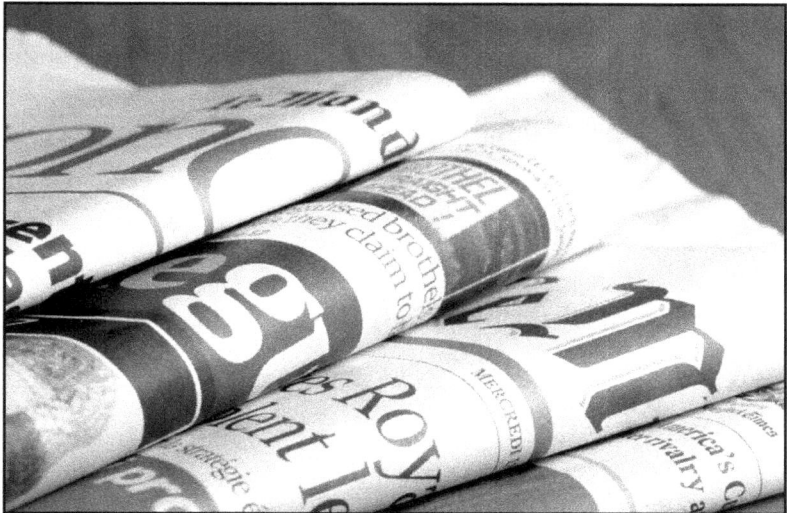

While many people will agree that our news is too depressing to read, it's still an invaluable source of information that can enhance you sense of criminal awareness.

• If someone approaches you in a threatening manner, try to keep them at a safe distance. If the situation and environment permits you to maintain a neutral zone, then by all means do so. The neutral zone is a safe distance that keeps you out of range of active engagement where you can be kicked, punched, grabbed, clubbed, slashed, or stabbed.

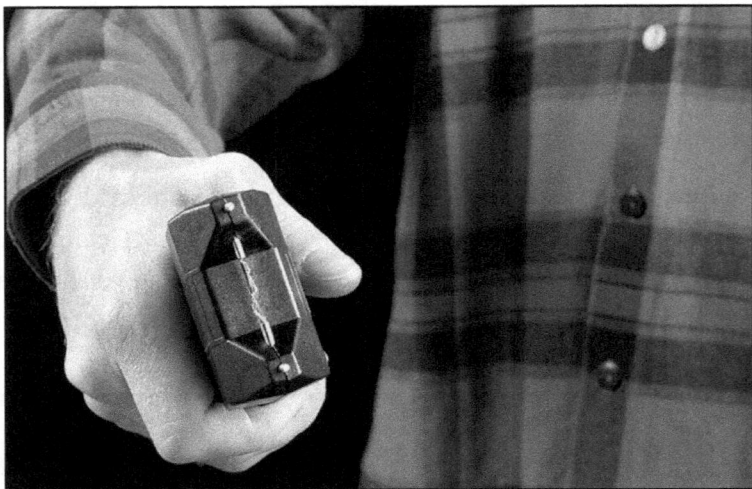

Stun guns use high voltage electricity to paralyze the body for a short period of time.

• Stun guns can be effective against criminals, but keep in mind that you have to be in very close proximity to the attacker in order to firmly press the contact probes against his body.

• To avoid theft, try to avoid using or displaying your smartphone in public places.

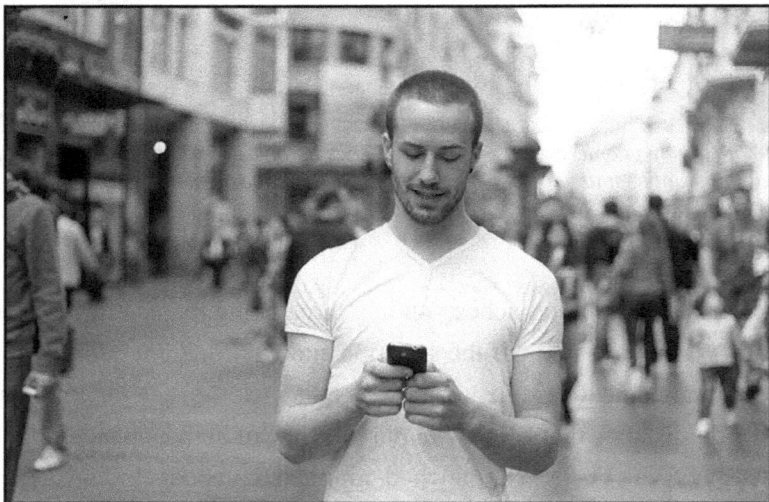

Just remember, criminals love to steal smartphones right from your hands.

• Remember to set your phone up to go into password protect mode when you take it with you.

• To avoid a backpack pickpocket carry your backpack in front of you while on the bus or subway. Be especially aware when using the escalator and stairs.

• According to FBI statistics, your chances of survival are dramatically reduced if you let your assailant take you from one crime scene location to another. Your best bet is to stand and fight for your life!

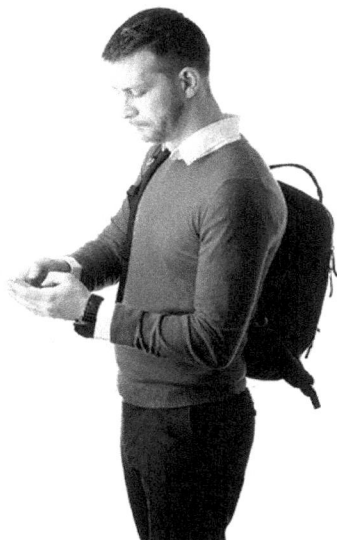

Criminals are well aware of the fact that 90% of the time they can find a cell phone or wallet inside the rearward facing pockets of a backpack.

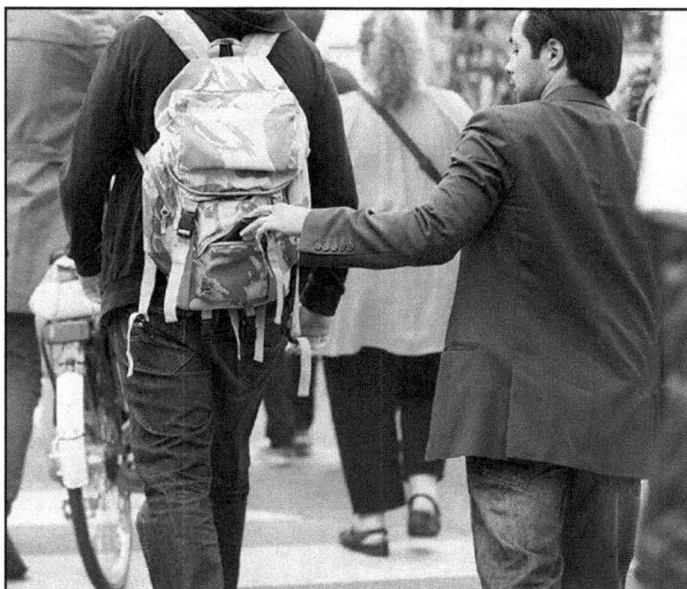

• Avoid putting vanity license plates on your car. They can bring attention to you and your family and possibly provoke problems on the road.

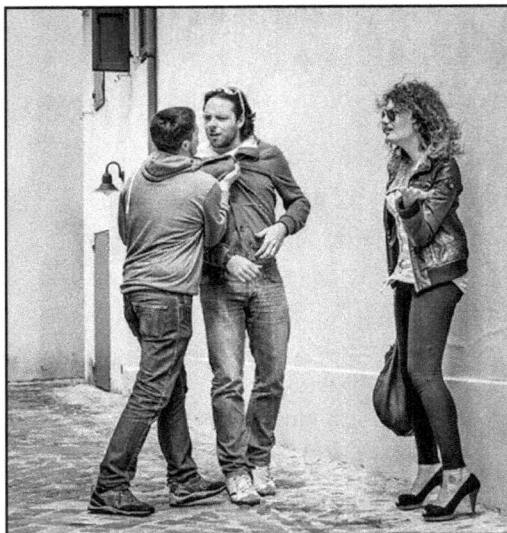

• Sit down with your spouse or significant other and discuss how the two of you will handle a criminal assault on the street. Discuss the possible strategies, tactics, and methods the two of you will use to deal with a threatening attacker.

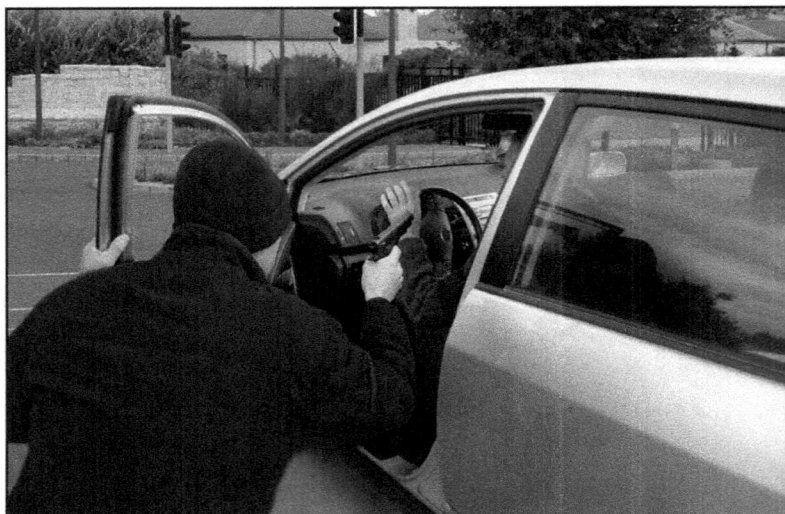

When faced with the carjacking scenario, stay calm and assess the situation to determine your best tactical response.

• Get into the habit of parking your car as close as you can to your destination and always make a mental note where you parked.

• When walking to your car, always be alert and suspicious of persons sitting idly in their cars.

• If there are suspicious people hanging around your car, do not approach it until they are gone.

• If you are the victim of a carjacking, remember that in most cases, the criminal is interested only in the vehicle. If he has a weapon, try to stay calm and avoid staring at him.

• When going to bars, restaurants, and nightclubs never leave your drink or cocktail unattended. Sexual predators are known to slip a "knockout drug" in your drink.

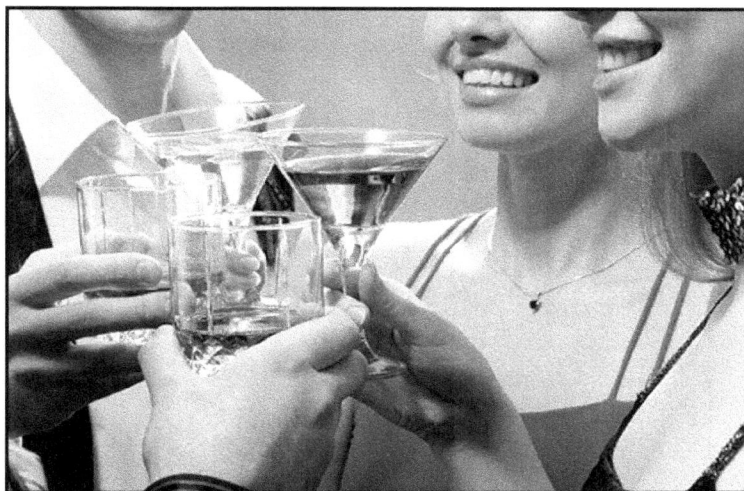

Never leave your drink unattended.

• Refrain from tasting anybody else's drink.

• According to the Justice Department, statistics indicate that a woman is less likely to be raped if she fights back against her attack-

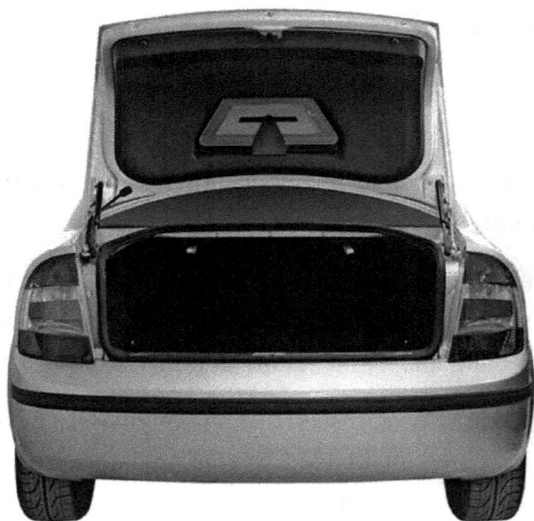

If ever you were forced into the trunk of a car, keep your cool and look for objects and opportunities to escape.

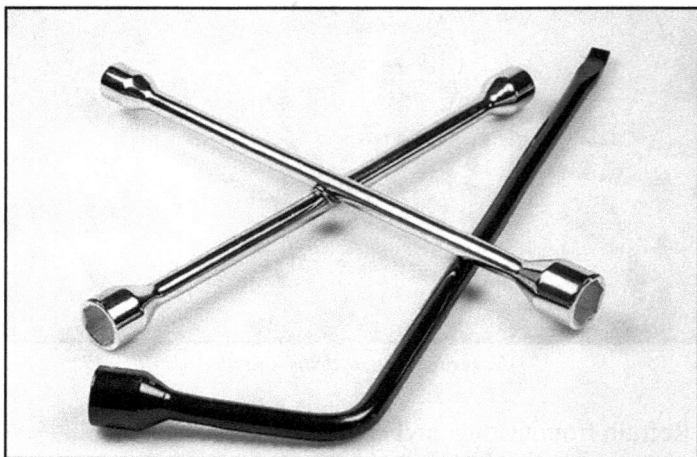

A lug wrench or tire iron can be used to help pry open the trunk. They also make great makeshift weapons to help fight your abductor.

er but she is more likely to get injured during the altercation.

• If you are abducted, and forced into the trunk of a car, remain calm and control your breathing. The important point is to keep your cool and assess the situation. If possible, try to maneuver yourself so you can kick out the back taillight. Once the taillight has been removed stick your arm out of the opening and wave your arms frantically to get attention from anyone on the road.

• Learn how to escape from the trunk of your own car. Make certain you know where the trunk release latch is located and that you are able to find it in the dark. For emergency situations, consider leaving a screwdriver, crowbar, or tire iron hidden in the trunk so you can use it to pry the latch open or use as a makeshift weapon to defend against your abductor.

• As soon as you enter your car, get into the habit of immediately locking the doors and driving away. Avoid the tendency to just sit and work when your car is parked. Avoid chatting on the phone, putting on makeup, reading, listening to music,etc. Criminal preda-

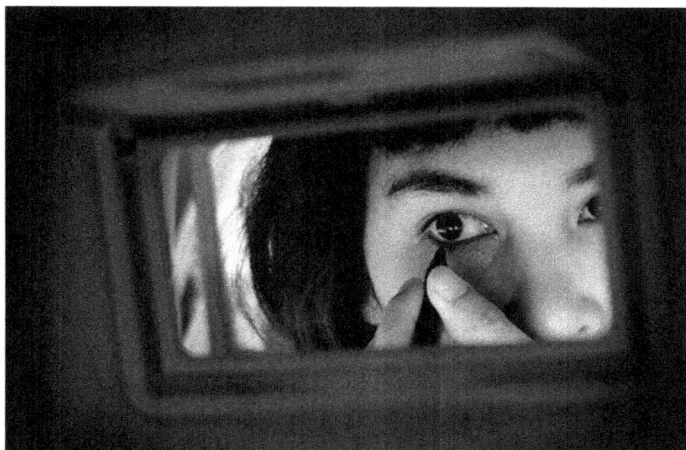

As soon as you enter your car, get into the habit of immediately locking the doors and driving away.

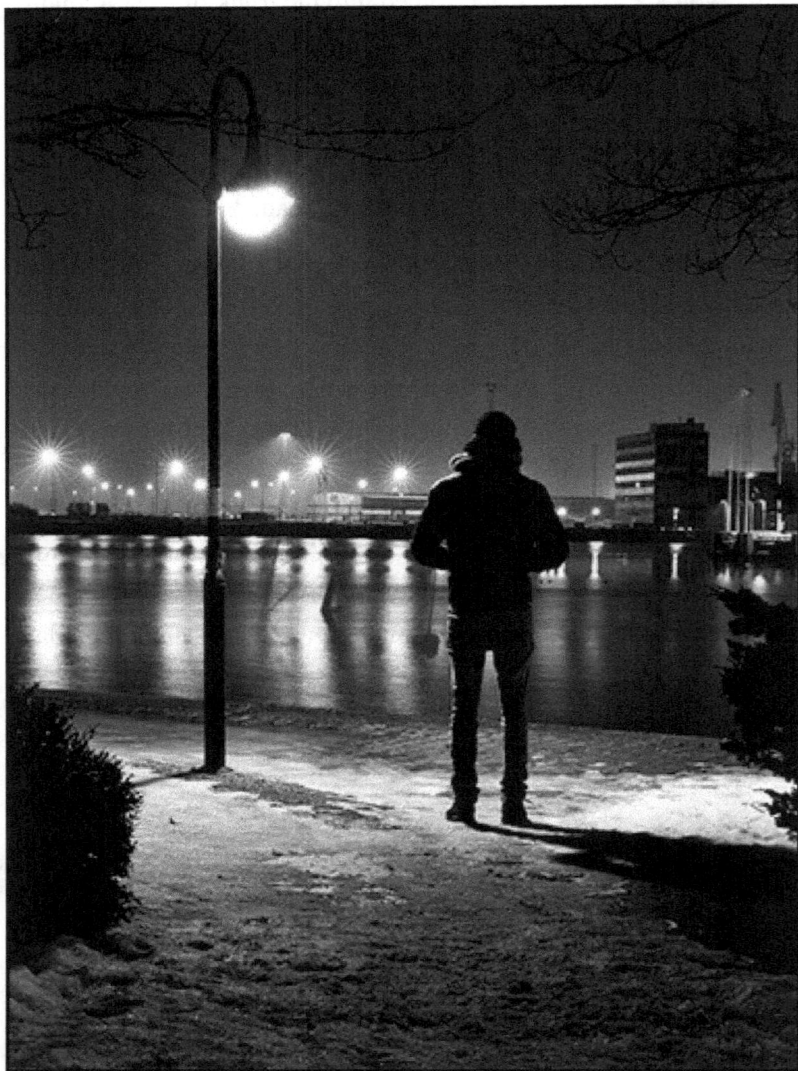

When someone confronts you on the street, try to maneuver yourself so the light source (i.e., street light, etc) is directly in the person's eyes.

tors look for opportunities when you are distracted in your car.

• If you are ever confronted by a stranger at night, try to maneuver yourself so the light source (i.e., street light, etc) is directly behind you and in your person's eyes.

• If you frequently walk the streets, consider carrying "throw money." Essentially, throw money is a decoy of cash that you would use in the event that you are mugged. The best way to prepare for this is to take a twenty dollar bill and fold it over a few one dollar bills. This gives the illusion that you have a big wad of cash. Keep the wad of cash held together with a strong rubber band or a cheap money clip. In the event that you are robbed, throw

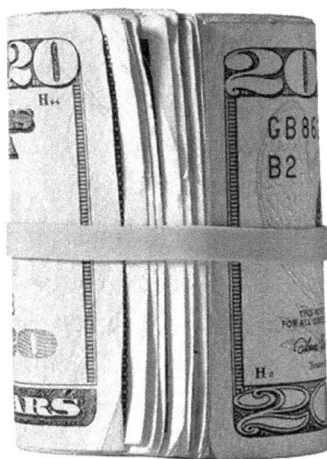

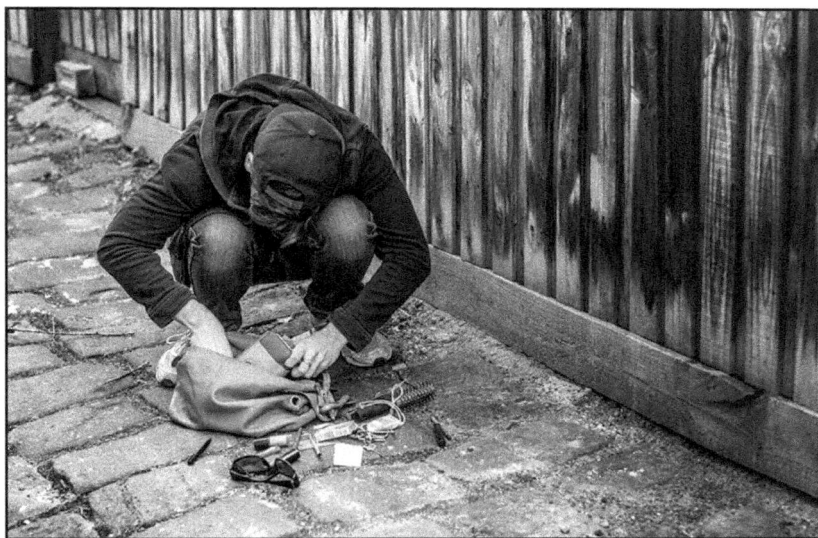

Throw money prevents the thief from taking all of your belongings, including your personal information.

the wad of cash in one direction and run the other way. The odds are the criminal will go after the cash instead of you.

• Always keep your throw money in a designated location such as a specific pant pocket or section of your purse. This will ensure that you can get to it quickly and easily.

• Consider carrying a kubotan self-defense key chain. The Kubotan is a devastating close-quarter self-defense weapon that can be used as both an impact tool and pain compliance device. This sturdy mini stick is approximately the size of a thick magic marker and it often has a keyring attached to its end. To learn more, see my book *Kubotan Power: Quick and Simple Steps to Mastering the Kubotan Keychain.*

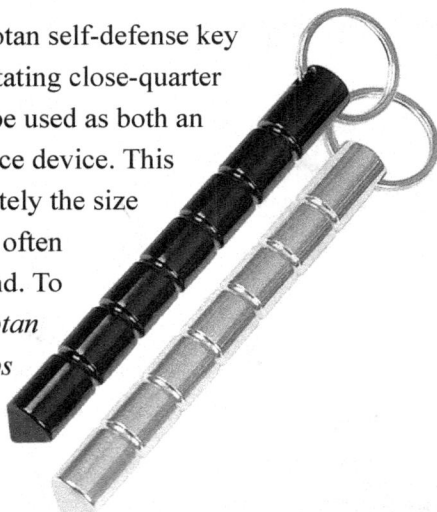

• If you are prohibited from carrying a kubotan, consider a tactical flashlight. As a matter of fact, the tactical flashlight is a great alternative to the kubotan because it functions as both an illumination tool and highly effective impact weapon.

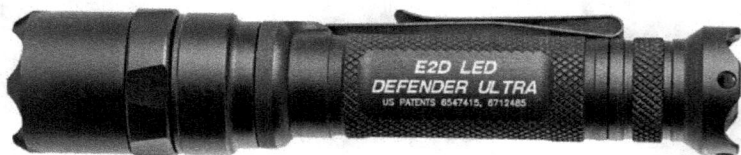

One of the best tactical flashlights on the market. The SureFire E2D LED Defender Ultra Flashlight.

• Always look under and inside your vehicle before you get too close to it.

• To improve your security and privacy on the road, consider having your car windows tinted.

• Don't use your car keys as an improvised striking weapon. You are better off using your natural body weapons such as: the heel of your palms, elbows, knees, etc.

• Never, ever recite your social security number in public, this includes banks. Instead, write it down on paper, hand it to the teller and then destroy it

.• Avoid wearing off-color or offensive t-shirts in public. While it might bring you a laugh or two, it can also bring trouble your way.

• After a self-defense altercation, there is always the possibility that you will have to deal with the police. Keep in mind that a police officers is permitted to approach you in a public place and request information. Furthermore, if the officer reasonably suspects that you are committing, have committed, or are about to commit a crime, he or she may detain you briefly for questioning.

• If a police officer reasonably suspects that you are armed and dangerous, he or she is permitted to frisk you without making an arrest. If while frisking you for weapons or evidence, the officer finds anything illegal, he can confiscate it and arrest you. What follows, are seven simple rules of conduct when confronted by the law.

1. Identify Yourself As The Victim - identify yourself as the victim and be prepared to show identification. Be careful and avoid quick or sudden movements when reaching for your wallet, and always try to keep your hands in plain view.

2. Be Polite And Respectful To The Officer - don't talk back to police officers, and always address them as either "sir" or "ma'am"

3. Watch What You Say - speak slowly and clearly, avoid using

profanity, sarcasm, and racial or derogatory remarks, and realize that what you say can be used against you.

4. Explain What Happened - clearly describe the sequence of events that led to the fight and if the assailant used a weapon.

5. Follow Orders - if the officer orders you to wait at a particular spot while he sorts out the matter, obey him.

6. Don't Get Angry - if you get angry or hostile with the police officers, you will land in jail.

7. Know Your Rights - finally, if you are arrested and taken into police custody, remember that you have the right to remain silent, obtain a lawyer, be informed of the charges against you, and have a judge decide whether you should be released on bail.

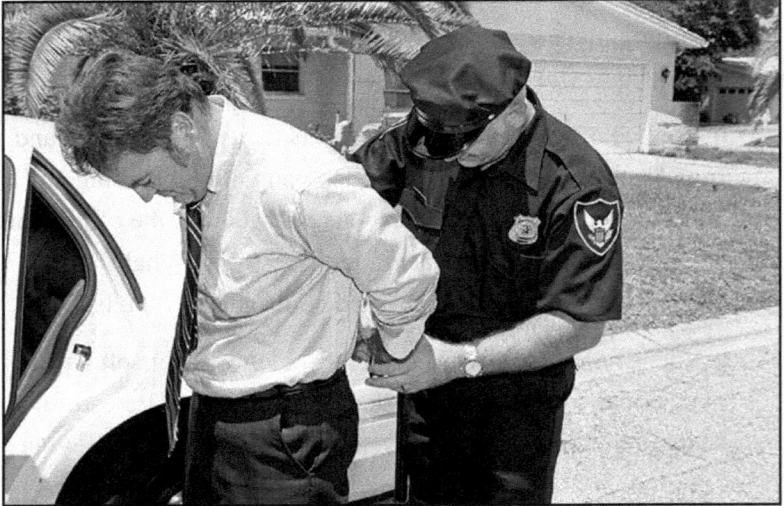

• Keep your life private, avoid unnecessary phone conversations in public places.

• When eating out at diners or restaurants, avoid sitting with your

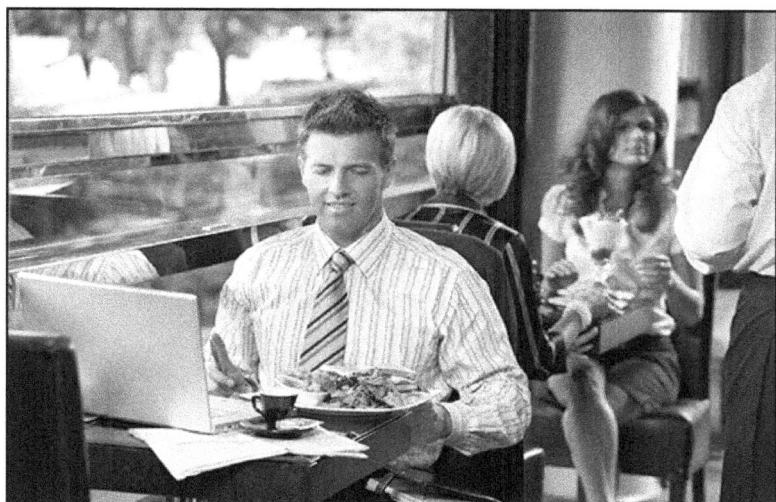

back to the door or entrance. Try to always sit with you back to the wall so you can see what is going on in your environment.

• When carrying a package or bag, try to carry it on the side furthest from the street. This will help reduce the chances of a "snatch and run" attempt.

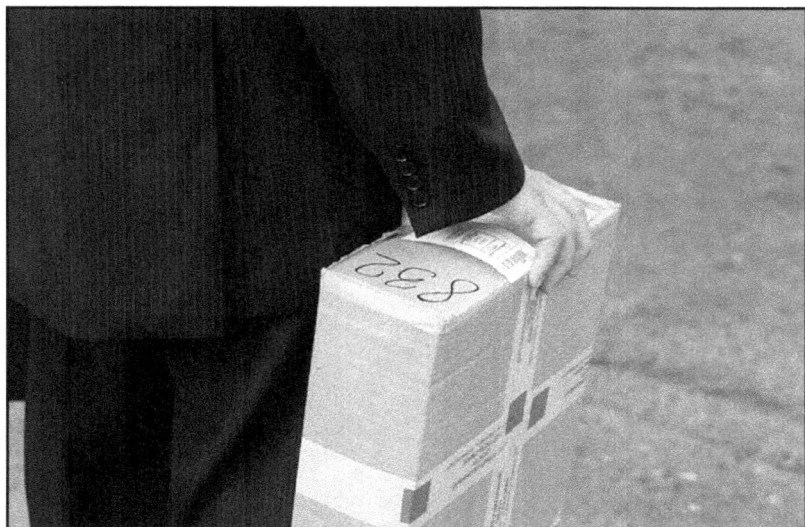

Self-Defense Tips and Tricks

• Avoid keeping valuables in your car, including GPS navigator, cellphones, tablets, computers, purses, briefcases, spare change, expensive sunglasses, etc.

• When parking your car in public places, consider leaving a man's hat in the back window or perhaps a baseball cap with a police insignia sewn on it.

• When meeting people for the first time, avoid conversations about religion, politics, and sex.

When driving, always keep a car length distance from the car in front of you so you can escape in an emergency.

• Keep your car well maintained and the gas tank at least half full to avoid getting stranded.

• When approaching your car, check your tire for flats. Criminals will often flatten your tires leaving you stranded and vulnerable to attack.

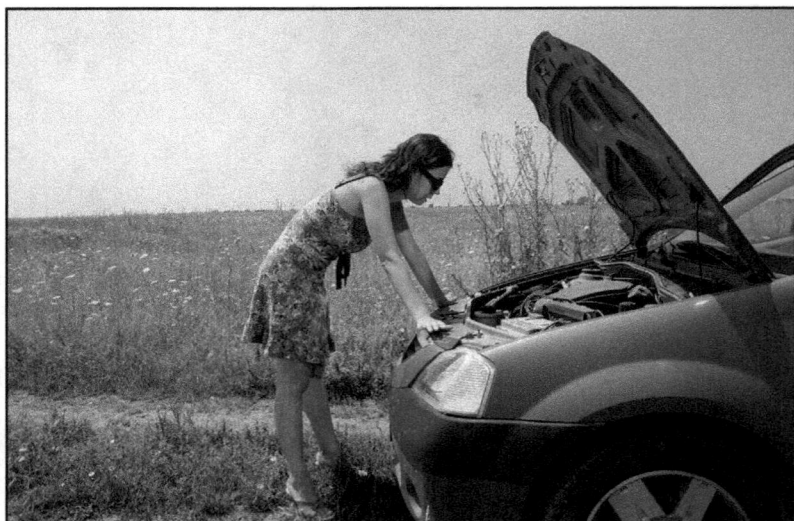

• Minimize the amount of money, credit cards and valuables you carry during the day.

• When walking, don't stop to talk with strangers. Remember, many street criminals will talk to their victims before they attack them.

• When walking outdoors, always have one hand free to defend yourself in the event of a surprise attack.

• When entering your car, get into the habit of locking your doors before you fasten your seatbelt.

• If your tire goes flat in a bad part of town, keep driving until you get to a safe location. Your life is more important than a damaged wheel or tire.

• Never, ever help a stranded motorist. Instead, use your cell phone and call for help.

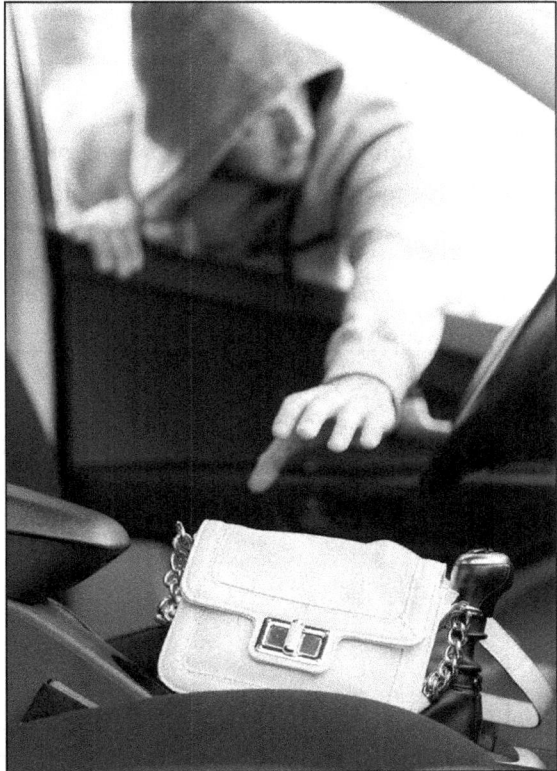

Always keep valuables secured in the trunk, not lying on the seat.

Self-Defense Tips and Tricks

- Do not pick up hitchhikers. The dangers should be obvious.

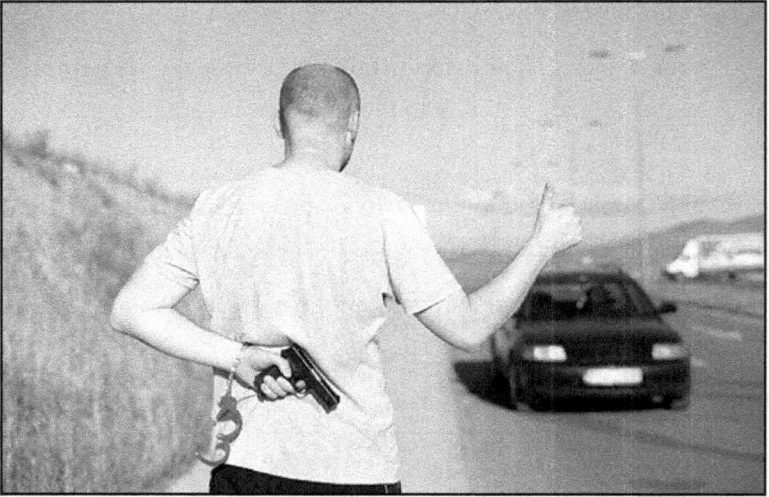

Don't feel obligated to pick up a hitchhiker just because you drove past him.

- If you think someone is following you in your car, do not drive home. Drive to the nearest police or fire station to get help.

- While eating out at restaurants, avoid hanging your purse or jacket over the back of your chair. Instead, keep your purse on your lap or between your feet.

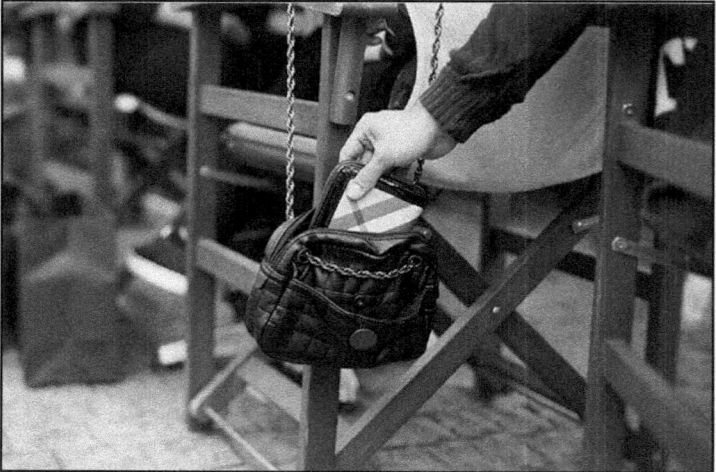

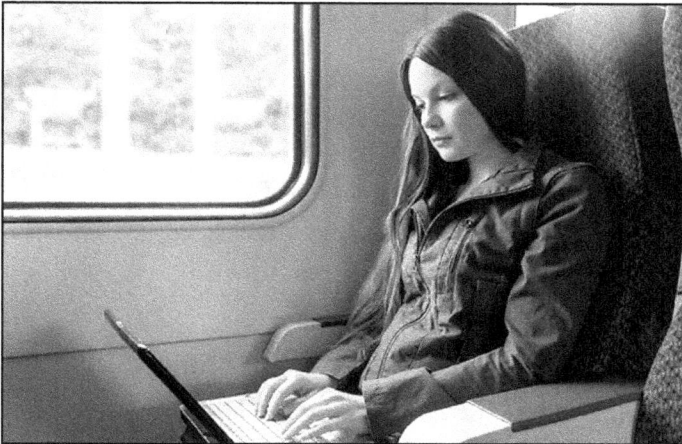

If you must work on your computer in public places, be certain strangers don't have visual access to your screen. Consider installing a privacy filter over your screen to keep your private data out of sight.

• Never allow a stranger to persuade or convince you to do something you really don't want to do. There is nothing wrong with the word, 'no."

• Never send and receive private information when using public Wi-Fi.

• Never leave your laptop, tablet, or smart phone unattended.

• When working on your computer, get into the habit of looking over your shoulder to see if anyone is watching you.

• If possible, avoid entering password information on public computers.

• Consider installing a privacy filter over your screen to keep your private data out of sight.

• If you must use the Internet on a public computer (library, computer store, Internet café, etc.), make certain to delete files and cookies and always clear your browsing history.

Self-Defense Tips and Tricks

• Before giving your credit card number to any commerce website, be absolutely certain it's a secure site.

• If you are purchasing an expensive gadget, try to avoid walking out of the store with the item in plain view. For example, if you are buying a new tablet or smartphone, consider carrying it out of the store in one of those tattered recyclable grocery bags. Avoid using store brand shopping bags, such as ones from Apple or Best Buy. Criminals will immediately target you!

• Avoid selling or purchasing items on websites such as Craigslist. However, if you must sell or purchase an item, consider the following:

1. If you're meeting the person, try to arrive at the designated location early and before they arrive. Try to park your car far enough away so the person won't easily see you but you'll be able to observe their behavior. Let your gut instincts decide if you should move forward with the meeting. If something seems wrong, for any reason, drive away immediately.

2. Always meet in a public place like a coffee shop, Café or restaurant.

3. Don't meet them alone. Bring a friend with you.

4. Never invite them to your home or meet at their place.

5. Always tell a family member or friend where you are going, who you are meeting, and exactly what you are doing.

6. Bring your cell phone with you.

7. Never give out personal or financial information for any reason.

8. If you are selling something, only accept cash. Never take a check!

Chapter Two
Home Protection

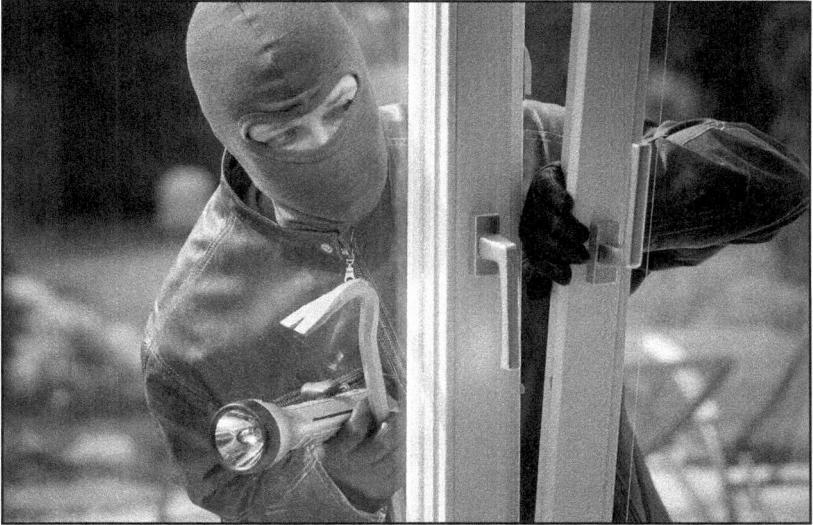

Self-Defense Tips and Tricks

• Keep doors and windows locked at all times.

• When sleeping, keep your bedroom doors locked.

• Never invite strangers into your home, no matter who they say they are.

• Never leave your garage door open or unlocked.

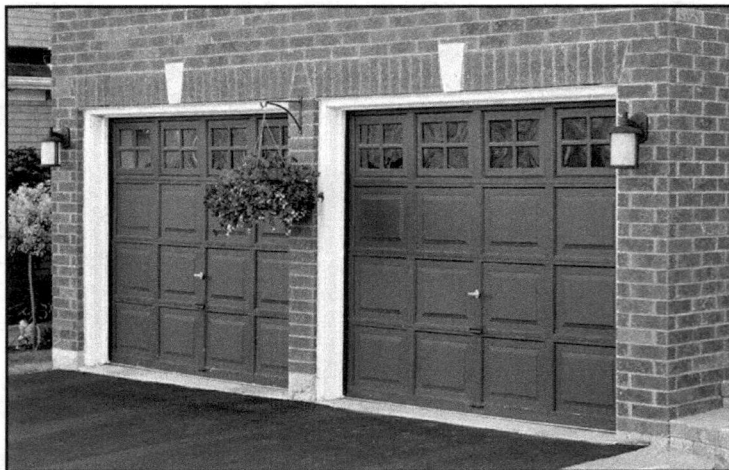

While it might be inconvenient, keep your garage doors closed at all times.

• Never enter your home if it shows any signs of possible entry. Go to a neighbor's and call the police.

• In the evening, leave interior and exterior lights on all night. Vary the lights you choose to leave on inside the house.

• Do not hide spare keys anywhere outside your home. This includes: door mats, flowerpots, and fake rocks.

• Do not open your door to strangers. If it's a law enforcement officer, ask to see identification. He or she will understand.

• If you own a dog, don't put him in harm's way and expect

them to attack an intruder. As a responsible pet owner, you have an obligation to protect him just like any other family member.

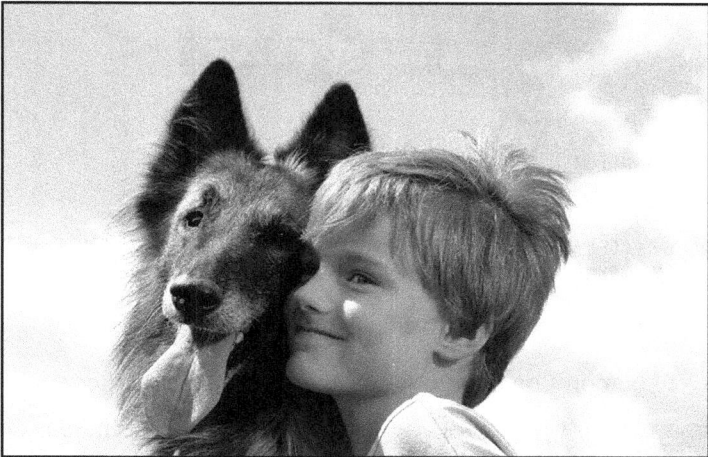

You have an obligation to protect your dog just like any other family member.

• Never keep large sums of money in your house.

• Don't rely solely on watchdogs. They can be, and have been, poisoned by intruders.

• To discourage burglars, keep your drapes, curtains, and blinds drawn in the evening.

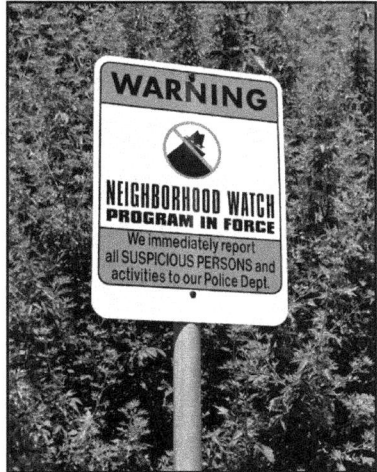

• Form and/or join neighbor-hood watch programs.

• Thieves can hide behind trees and shrubs, so keep the trees and shrubbery around windows and doors well trimmed.

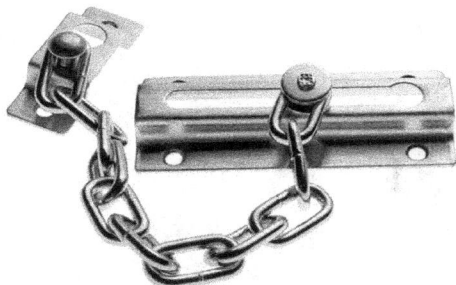

Security chains on doors will not keep a power assailant from forcing his way into your home. Don't rely on them!

• Do not rely on security chains on doors.

• If you don't own a home alarm system, consider keeping your car keys next to your bed. For example, if you suspect there is an intruder in your home, press the panic button on your key fob. In most cases, the car alarm will startle the burglar.

• If you keep firearms in your home, keep them in a burglarproof safe when you are away. Keep them away from children at all times. Be trained extensively in safe handling and self-defense procedures. Armed novices are dangerous to themselves and others.

• Secure sliding glass exterior doors with bar braces. Or use a wooden or metal rod in the track on sliding patio doors to prevent them from being opened.

• Make certain all window screens are properly latched.

• Install heavy duty window frames.

• Never give your keys to service people, i.e., carpenters, painters, repairmen, etc.

• Report any voyeurs to the police immediately.

• Never put your name and address on your key ring.

• A good way to prevent burglars and peeping toms from peering into your windows is to plant thorny shrubs beneath the ground floor windows.

• Use only your initials and last names on mailboxes.

• Put dead bolts on all doors and make certain they all have a minimum 1-inch throw. Never rely on spring bolts. They can be jimmied very easily.

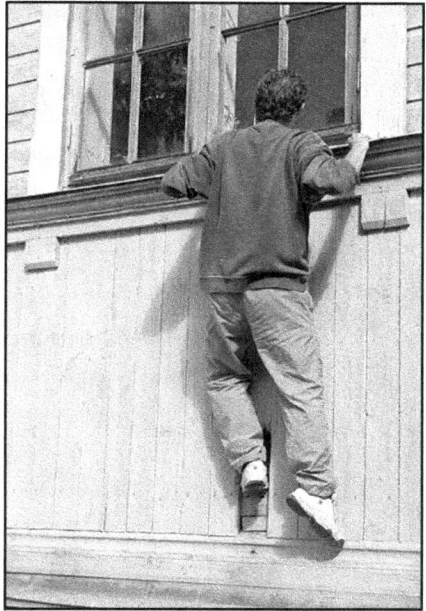

• Be suspicious of all unanticipated delivery persons.

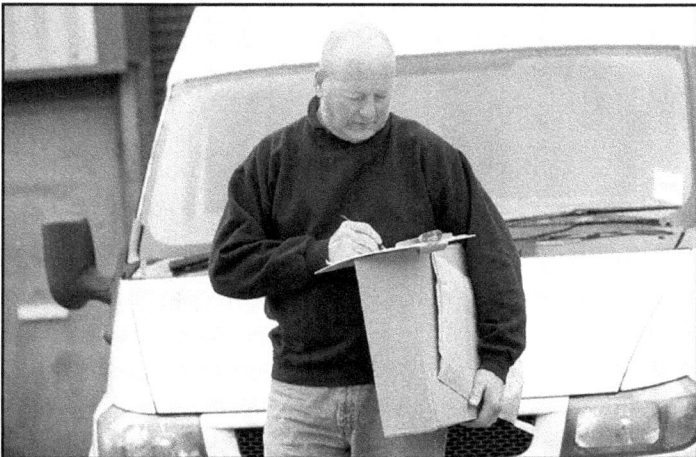

There is nothing wrong with being suspicious of all unanticipated delivery persons.

Self-Defense Tips and Tricks

• If you can afford it, consider installing a security alarm system in your house. Studies do show that robbers leave faster and take less of your property if your alarm goes off.

• While burglar alarms or electronic security systems are effective, don't rely solely on them. They are not a guarantee that burglars will not enter your home and they can be disarmed. Further, they simply serve as a warning of danger. You must have a planned and effective response to the danger itself. Sit down with your family and design a few strategic plans to handle various home emergencies (e.g., burglary, fire, flood, etc.).

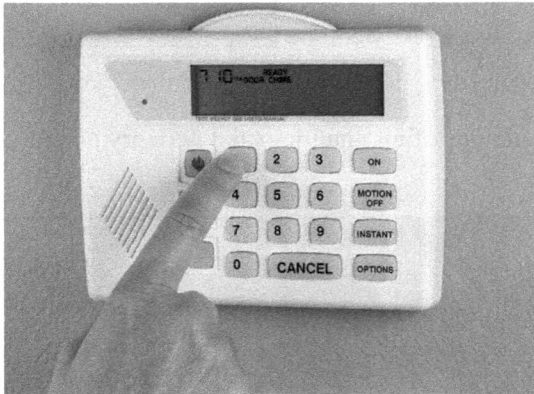

Security alarms only serve as a warning of danger, they do not eliminate the threat.

• Make certain all exterior doors are solid with 1 3/4-inch hardwood.

• Install a wide-angle viewer in your front door.

• Install heavy duty door locks with strike plates.

- If you live in an apartment building, avoid using the stairs.

- When moving into a new house or apartment, install new locks.

- Never leave notes on your front door. It's an invitation to a burglar.

- If you live in an apartment building with an elevator, test the emergency button. If it stops the elevator, don't use it if you are in an elevator with a suspicious person or an attacker. You don't want to be stuck between floors with your assailant.

- Never leave ladders unchained outside your home, and never leave them up against the house.

- If under attack in an elevator, push the buttons for all the floors. Chances are you'll stop on a landing where someone will be able to help you or where you can attempt to flee.

- Always keep a flashlight close to your bed or night stand.

- Consider posting a theft deterrent sign in the front of your home, such as "trespassers will be shot", "guard dog on premises", "this property monitored by video surveillance."

- Routinely check the locks on all the doors around your house.

- If ever you are attacked in your apartment hallway, avoid

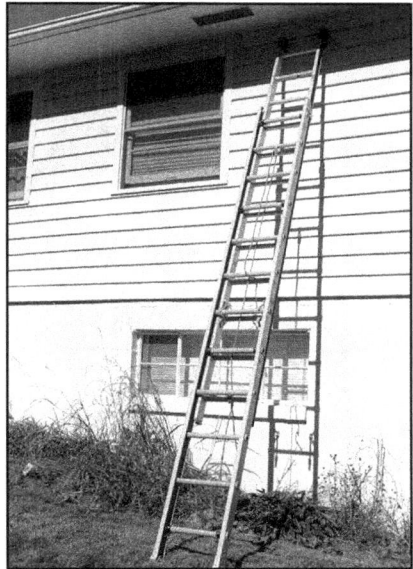

Never leave a ladder up against your house. You are just asking for trouble.

yelling "help!" Instead scream "fire!" Most tenants will rush out of their apartments.

• To help the police or fire department identify your home quickly, make certain your house number is clearly visible to the street.

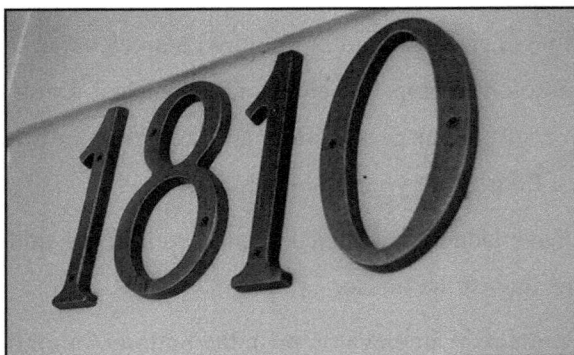

In the event of an emergency, make certain your house number is clearly visible from street.

• To make your home look occupied, keep the lawn sprinkler on when you leave the house.

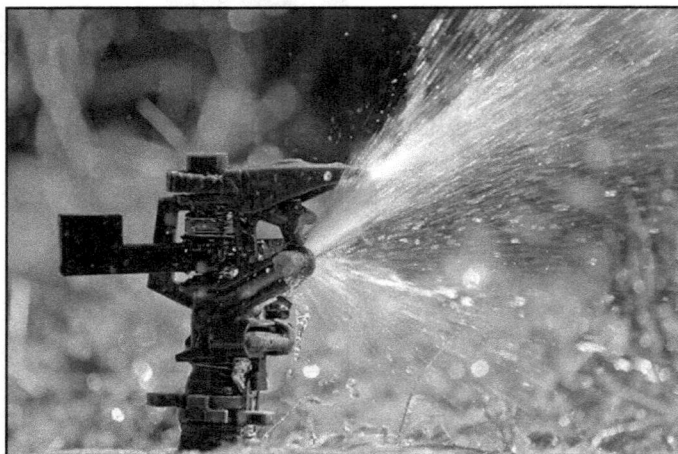

Something as simple as a running sprinkler will give the impression that your home is occupied.

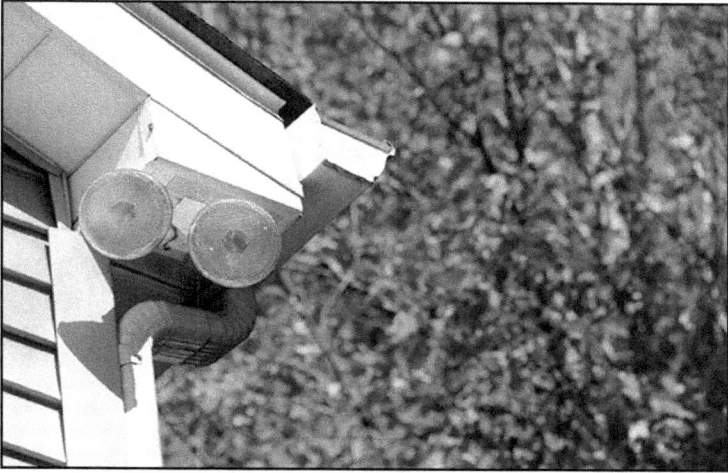

Floodlights are an excellent deterrent to criminals.

• To discourage prowlers, consider installing floodlights in your backyard.

• Don't leave messages on your front door; they tell burglars that you're not home.

• Keep your garage door closed and cover garage windows to keep burglars from looking in.

• Get into the habit of closing the garage door when you get home before exiting your car. Also, consider installing a large, full length mirror where you park, so you can see if someone enters the garage when you pull in.

• Teach family members to make it a nightly routine to check the locks before going to bed.

• Avoid storing wood near the side of your home. Burglars can use it as step ladder to a window.

• Consider placing a security alarm decal or sign in front of your home. Such items can help deter thieves from breaking into your home. Even if you don't have a security system, put it up anyway. Regularly check to make sure the sign is clearly visible and is not covered up by shrubs or knocked over by pets or lawn equipment.

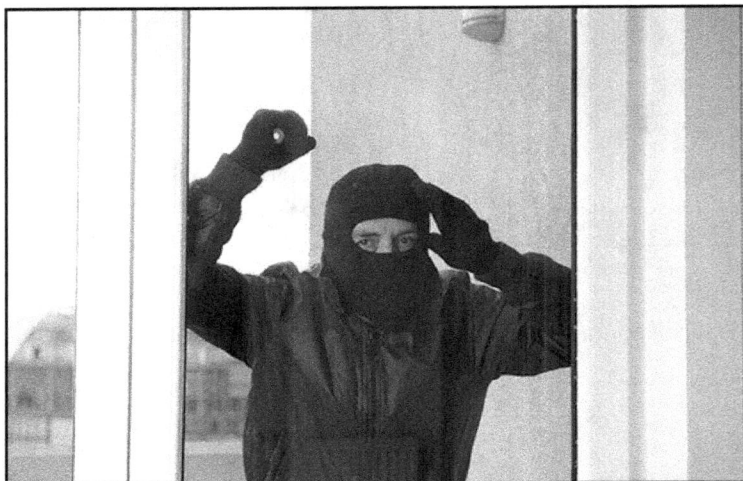

Don't make it easy for a burglar. Place window treatments on all of your windows.

Try "casing" your own home by attempting to gain access to your place when the doors and windows are locked.

• If you ever confront a burglar in your home, stay calm. Do not try to stop him. If possible, try to escape to safety.

• If you have a safe in your home, avoid hiding your keys or combination number in obvious places.

• Write down the license number of suspicious vehicles that drive through your neighborhood.

• Know your neighbors. Know who belongs in your neighborhood and who doesn't. Get to know your neighbors' cars.

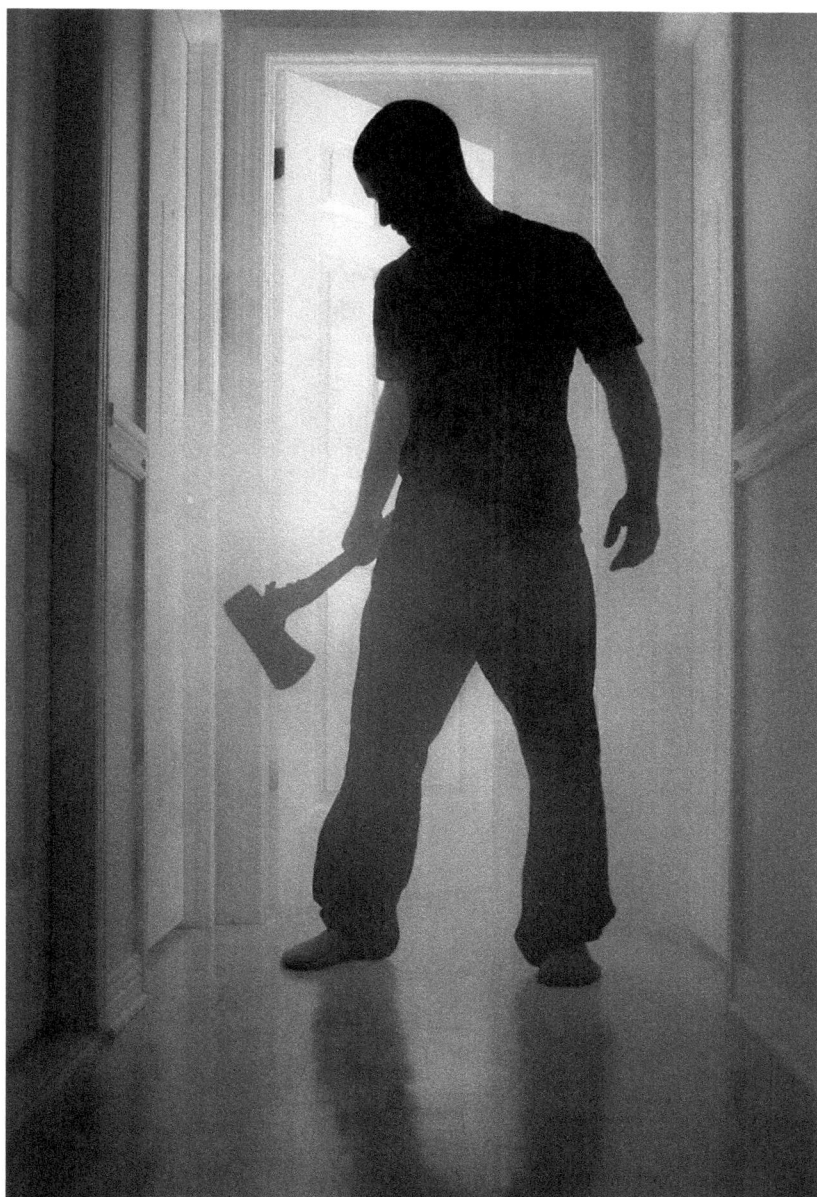

If you ever confront a burglar in your home, stay calm. Do not try to stop him. If possible, try to escape to safety.

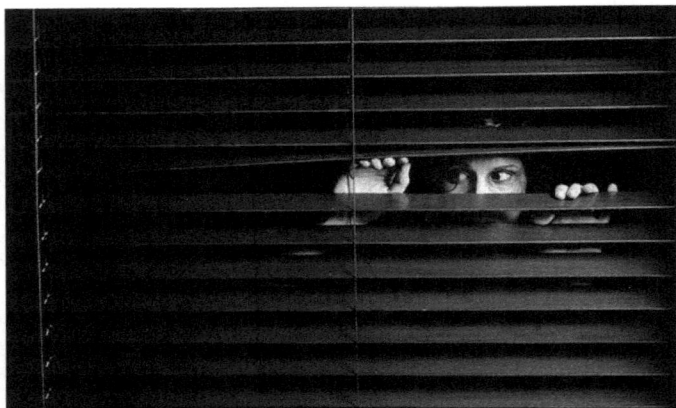

Be familiar with who belongs in your neighborhood and who doesn't.

• Get into the habit of turning the volume of your phone's ringer down so someone outside can't hear them ring. You don't want them to know that you are not home.

• When leaving your home, consider leaving a $10 bill in plain view (perhaps on a on a table in the foyer). If you come home and its missing, chances are you had a break in while you are away or perhaps someone is still in the house.

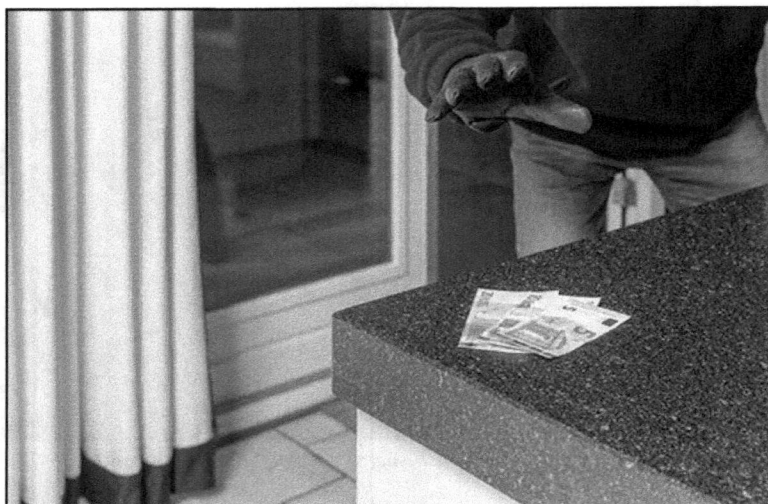

• Avoid having a horizontal mail slot installed in your front door. Mail slots tend to weaken the structural integrity of your door and will make it easier for criminals to force his way in.

• When installing a security keypad on your wall, make certain it is not visible from the front door.

• To prevent access to your home, cut back large tree limbs that hang over the roof.

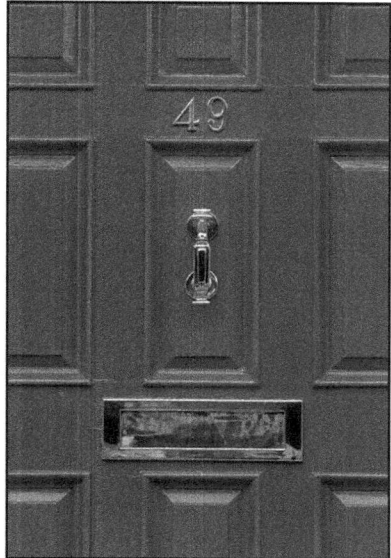

A mail slot might be convenient but it weakens the structural integrity of your front door.

• Never use geo-location on social media websites like Facebook.

• Avoid keeping your car keys and house keys on the same ring. Parking lot attendants can duplicate your house keys.

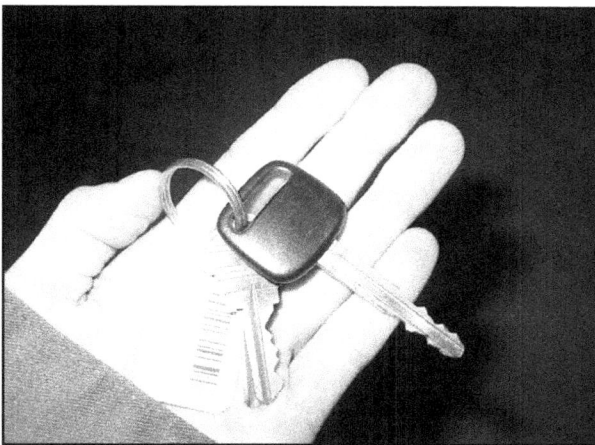

Remember to keep your car and home keys separate.

59

• Unless it's absolutely necessary, don't let contractors have full access to your house. For example, close doors to rooms that are not part of the home repair project.

• If you are having contractors work at your home, ask them to provide portable restrooms for outside jobs, or give them directions to the closest gas station.

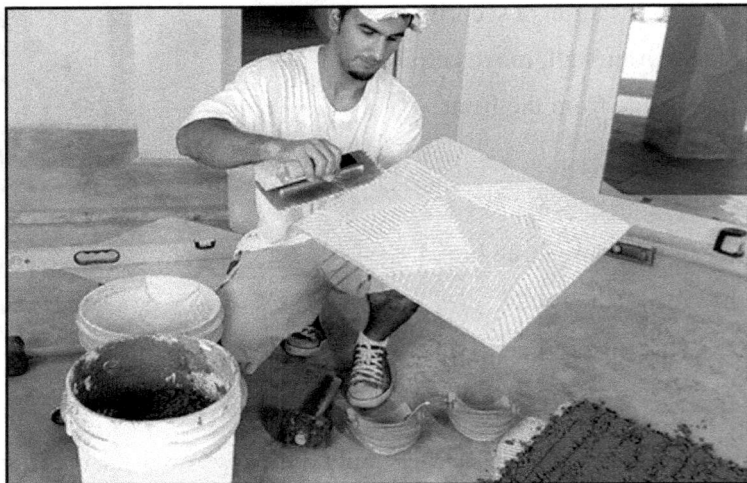

Unless it's absolutely necessary, don't let contractors have full access to your house.

• Never show pictures of expensive gifts or possessions you own on social media sites.

• Remember to lock crawl spaces and shed doors.

• During the holidays, avoid displaying holiday gifts in view of your windows or doors.

• Establish a safe room in your home. A "safe room" is a place where family members can escape from the intruder and wait for the police to arrive. Most people choose a particular bedroom in their house. Be certain there is a working telephone (preferably a cellular phone , in case the land line has been cut) in the safe room so you can contact an emergency dispatcher during a threatening encounter.

• If you think there is an intruder in your home, call the police immediately - even if you aren't absolutely certain. It is better to be safe than sorry.

• Install outside security lighting at every access door to your home.

• Use exterior lighting with motion sensors for the yard and driveway. Burglars are less likely to try breaking into your home if the light comes on.

• When taking out the trash, avoid leaving packaging for expensive purchases on the curb. For example, throwing out the box for your new computer or flat screen TV and displaying it out in the open lets everyone driving by know that you have expensive items in

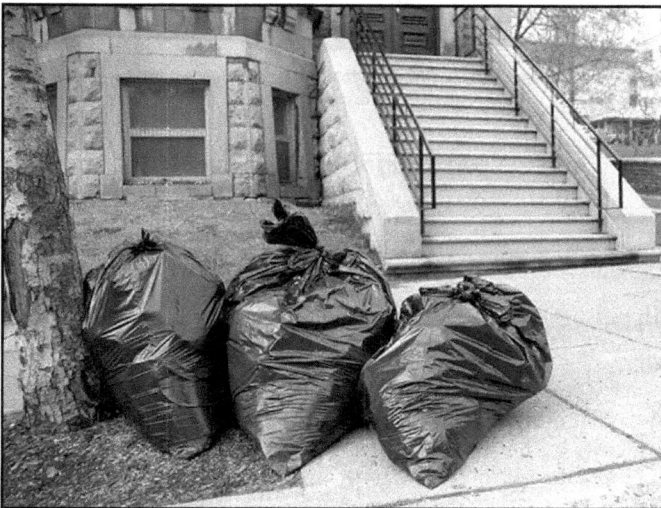

Leaving packaging for expensive purchases in contractor bags.

your home. Consider keeping the boxes for future storage, or breaking down the packaging and placing it inside contractor bags.

• Don't arm a criminal with information about your family. Avoid placing those family stick figure bumper stickers on back of your car.

• If possible, avoid glass panel or hollow-wood exterior doors. A determined criminal will blast right through them.

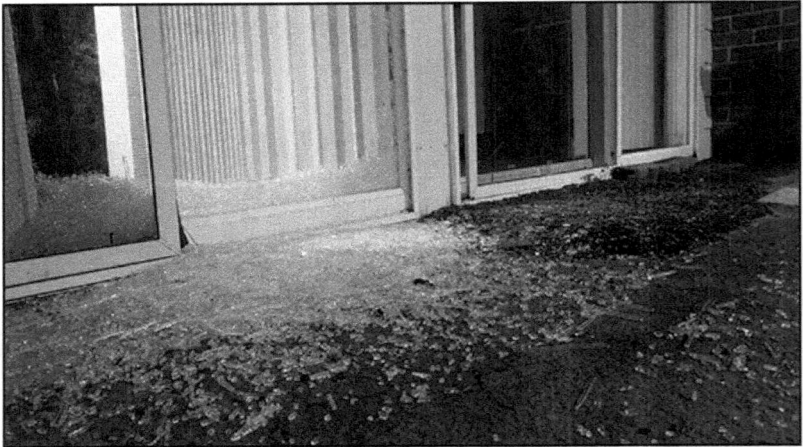

Criminals easily blast through exterior glass panel doors.

• Never provide personal information over the phone to a stranger.

• If you receive an obscene phone call, a threat, or other harassing call, get off the phone immediately and call the police and phone company.

• Avoid listing your name and home number in a directory.

• Keep your phone close to your bed. Beware of burglars who often take phones off the hook after entering a home to keep you from calling the police on your upstairs or bedroom phone. Have a different line installed in your bedroom or use your cell phone.

• Learn to operate and dial your phone in the dark.

• Consider purchasing Caller-ID to deter prank or problem callers.

• Have your telephone lines buried to prevent a would-be intruder from cutting the line.

• Keep logs of all threatening or problem calls you receive.

• Keep a list of important numbers by your phone, i.e., police, emergency ambulance, hospital, fire station, doctor, neighbors, close relatives, etc.

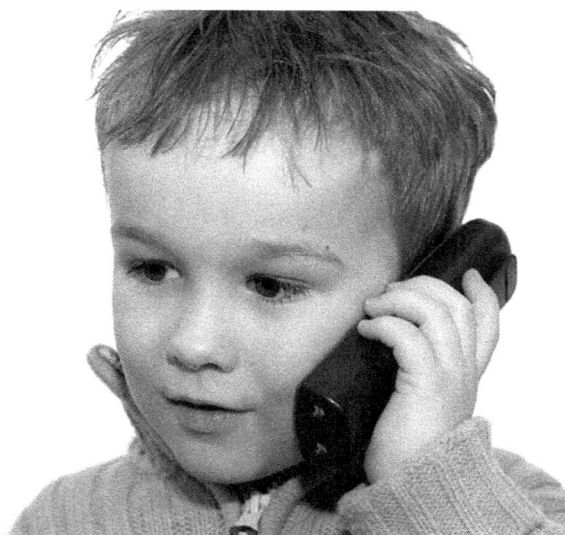

• If you let your children answer phones, instruct them not to give information to any strangers.

• Train your children in the use of the phone for emergency dialing and requests for help.

Self-Defense Tips and Tricks

• Avoid answering telephone survey questions.

• If you have an answering machine, do not let your child leave the outgoing message.

• Never answer your home telephone with your name.

• If you are thinking of owning a gun for home protection, you need to ask yourself these important questions before visiting the gun shop.

1. Do you abuse alcohol or use drugs? If so what kind?

2. Are you hot tempered?

3. Could you take the life of another person?

4. Do you experience long periods of depression?

5. Do you live alone?

6. Do children live in your household?

7. Why do you want to own a firearm?

8. Have you ever shot a gun?

9. Are you a disorganized person?

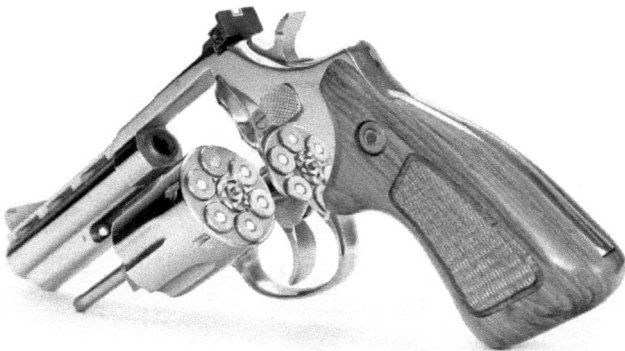

10. Are you clumsy or accident prone?

11. Are you willing to take the time to obtain the knowledge and learn the skills and attitude needed to handle firearms safely?

• Don't even think about owning a gun unless you have successfully completed a firearm safety course, been extensively trained in its use, and have developed the necessary confidence and proficiency.

• Safe gun handling is your responsibility, and safety must always be your concern. To ensure the safe use of any firearm, always follow these four primary safety rules:

1.   Always assume a firearm is loaded;

2.   Always point a firearm in a safe direction;

3.   Always be certain of your target;

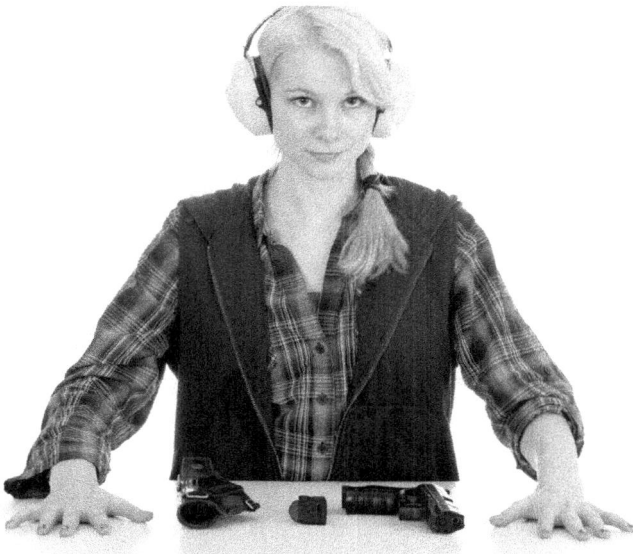

Gun ownership is not for everyone, however if you do decide to own a gun for home protection, be certain to complete a firearm safety course.

4. Never put your finger on the trigger until you are ready to shoot.

• If you own a firearm for home protection, make certain it is easily accessible in an emergency situation. Consider keeping a push button strong box by your bed and be capable of quickly opening it in the dark.

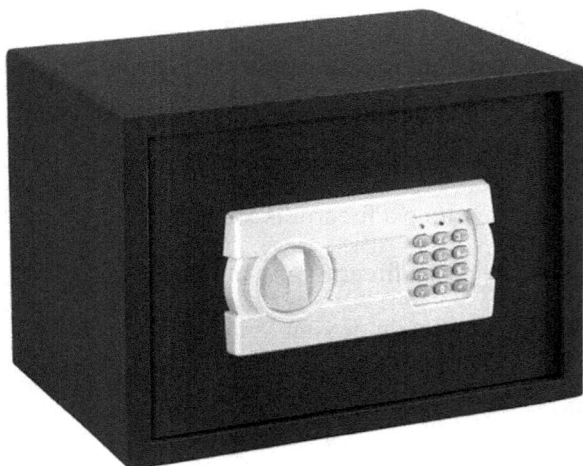

Strong boxes offer decent security for your handgun.

• Shooting a gun is just like any other physical skill that requires practice to become proficient. The firing range is the best place to effectively learn how to use a firearm in a self-defense situation. If you do own a firearm and plan on using it in an emergency situation, then it's your personal responsibility to visit the firing range on a consistent basis. This is especially important for law enforcement officers.

• Before you purchase a firearm, it is your responsibility to understand and obey the various laws governing its use, possession and transportation. Such laws vary from state to state, so learn the ones that apply to you and your community. Your local police or sheriff's department can help you.

• If you own a gun for home protection, consider utilizing a tactical flashlight in conjunction with your weapon. A tactical flashlight is important for the following reasons:

1. To positively identify your target.

2. To temporarily blind your assailant as you fire at him.

3. To provide a source of illumination to see where you are going in the dark.

4. To illuminate your assailant for accurate shooting.

5. To use as a striking make-shift weapon when lethal force is not warranted or justified.

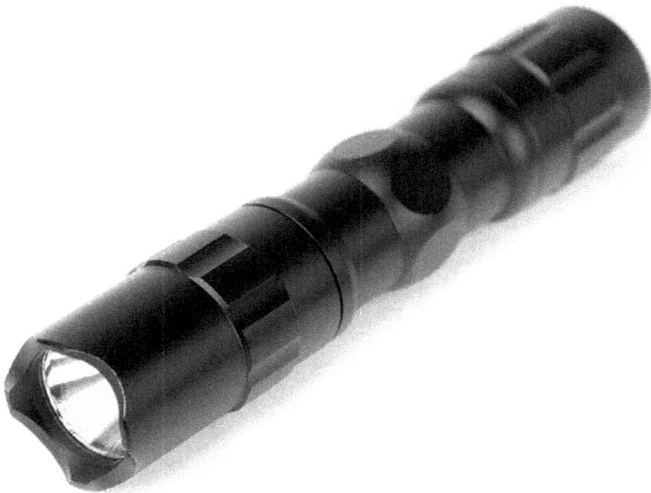

Pictured here, a tactical flashlight.

Self-Defense Tips and Tricks

Chapter Three
Workplace Safety

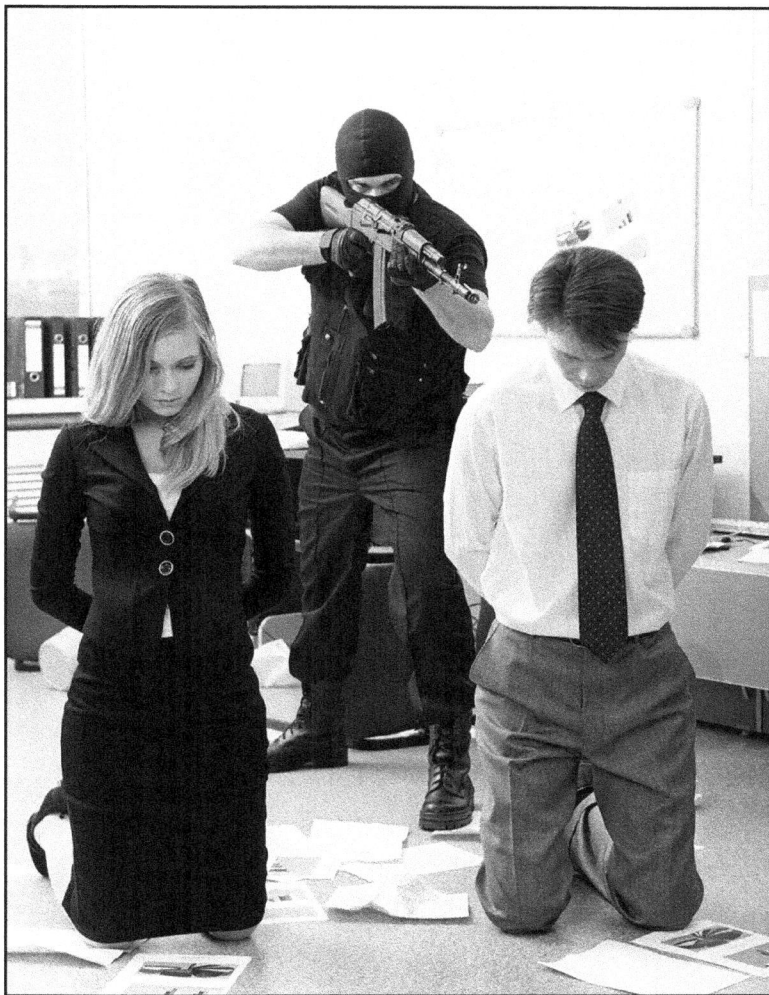

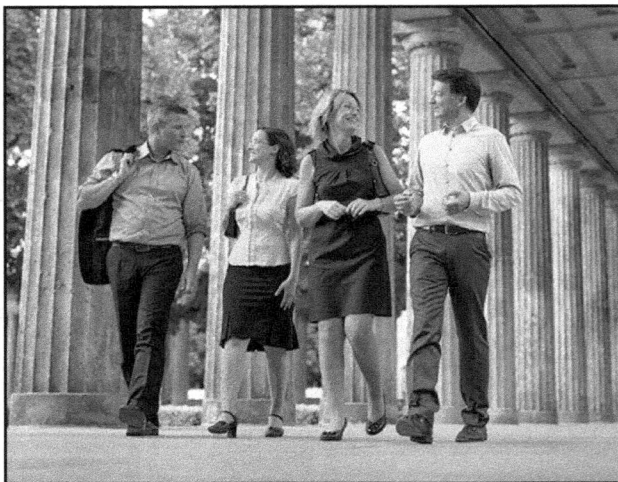

Try to encourage your co-workers to leave together when work is over.

• When work is over, try to encourage your co-workers to leave together.

• Be aware of the people who work in your office or building.

• Always lock your wallet or purse in your drawer.

• When exiting your building, get into the habit of looking in all directions as you exit.

• Know where all the various fire escapes are located in your building.

• Avoid having your name or title displayed at your company parking lot.

• Avoid working late in the office.

• Always have your car key in your hand when leaving the building.

• If you are going to work late, try to do it with another employee.

70

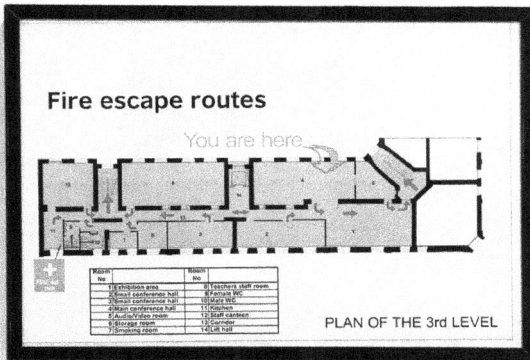

Fire escape routes

PLAN OF THE 3rd LEVEL

Do you know where all of the fire escapes are located in your office building?

• If you notice any suspicious people in your building or office, notify security or police.

• Avoid taking the stairs in your building.

• Be particularly cautious in deserted rest rooms.

• If you are leaving work in the evening, ask the security guard to escort you to your car.

• Ask your company's human resources division to arrange a self-defense seminar for all of the employees.

• When using the elevator, make it a habit to stand next to the control panel. If you are attacked, press all the buttons so the elevator will stop at every floor, giving you the opportunity to quickly escape.

• Be careful who you socialize with at work. Avoid disclosing too much personal information to any of your coworkers. If possible, try to socialize with people who share your values.

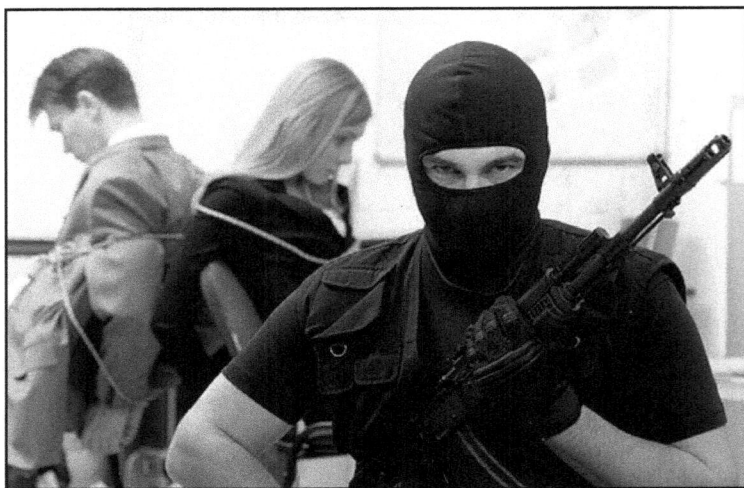

Surviving an Active Shooter Situation

• It is important to first understand the definition of an active shooter. According to the Department of Homeland Security, an active shooter "is an individual actively engaged in killing or attempting to kill people in a confined and populated area, typically through the use of firearms."

• Some characteristics of an active shooter situation are: victims are selected at random, the event is unpredictable and usually evolves quickly and law enforcement is usually required to end the situation. Some of the most common motives of an active shooter include: revenge, anger, ideology, and mental illness.

• During an active shooter situation, you only have three possible options:

1.   **Escape from the shooter**. If possible, leave your possession behind and quickly escape from the gunman. Look for

escape routes, these are the various avenues or exits that allow you to safely flee from the threatening situation. Some escape routes are windows, fire escapes, doors, gates, escalators, fences, walls, bridges, and staircases.

When approaching the police, remain calm and collected. Avoid screaming, yelling or crying. Keep your hands raised up and avoid any sudden movements. Do not approach the police with items in your hands such as briefcases, tablets, bags, jackets, etc. Drop them to the floor immediately and walk calmly to the officers.

If you do manage to escape from the shooter, cooperate with police and be prepared to give them the following information:

- The last location of the shooter.

- The number of shooters

- Physical description of the active shooter.

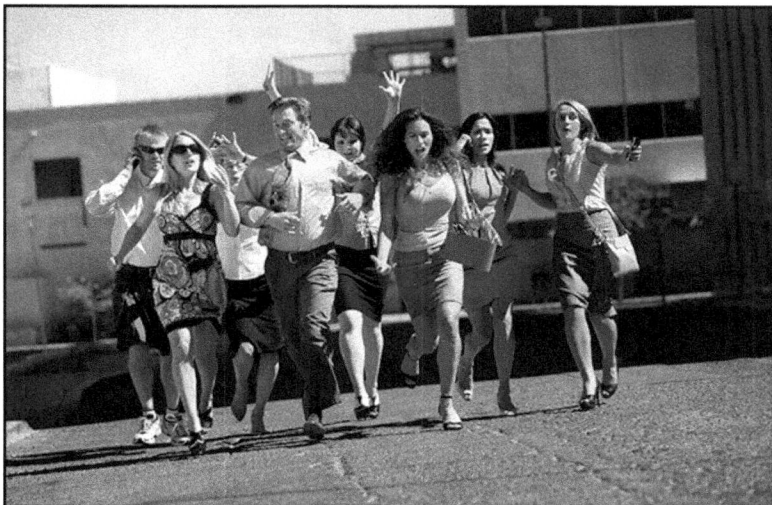

Do not approach the police with items in your hands. Drop them to the floor immediately and walk calmly to the officers.

- Type of weapons (i.e., handgun, rifle, shotgun, bomb, etc).

- The amount of ammunition (how many rounds or ammo?).

- The number and location of people still left behind.

- The number and location of possible injured or dead.

- The demeanor of the active shooter(s).

- Possible injuries sustained by the active shooter.

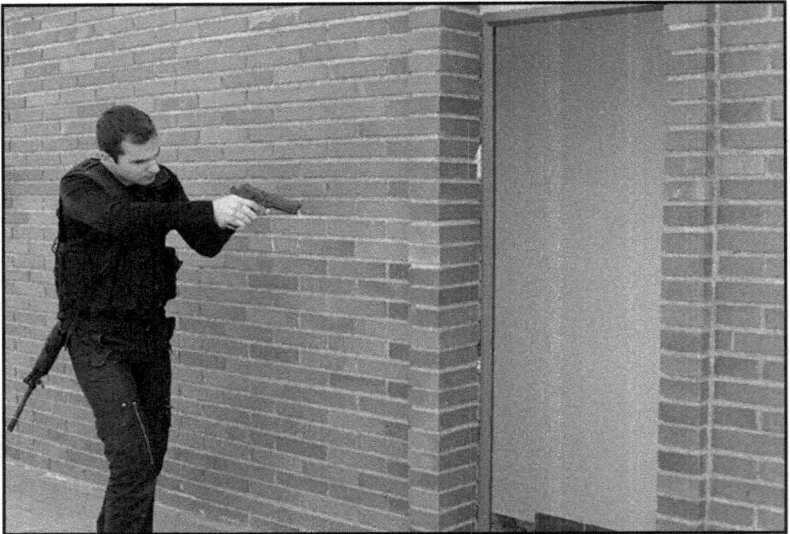

When evacuating the building, make certain your hands are visible to the police. Remember, they have no idea who is a victim and who is the active shooter.

2. **Hide from the shooter.** This means you will need to hide from the shooter's using a position of concealment. First, turn off radios or other devices that emit sound. If possible, block entry to your hiding place and lock the doors. Positions of concealment are various locations or objects that allow you to temporarily hide from the active shooter. Positions of concealment are most commonly used to evade engagement with your assailant(s) and they permit you to attack with

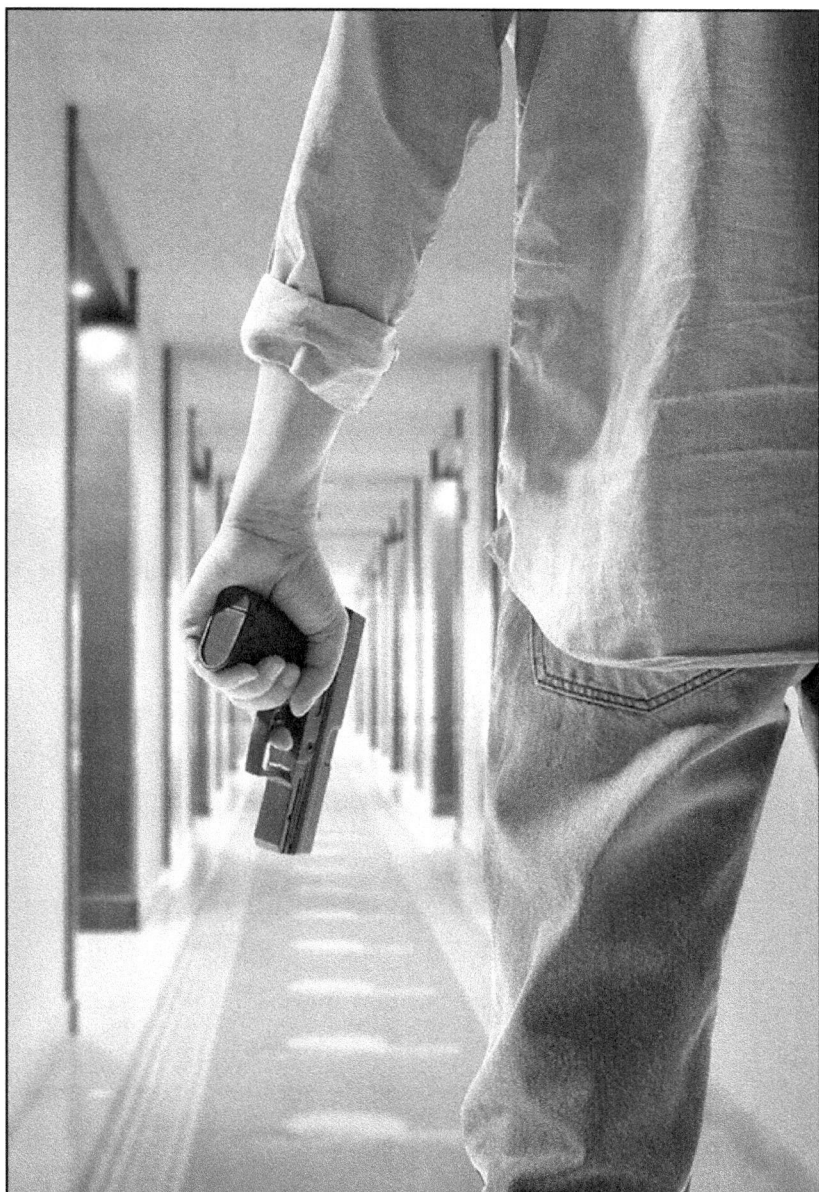

Active shooters generally don't have a pattern or method for selection of their victims.

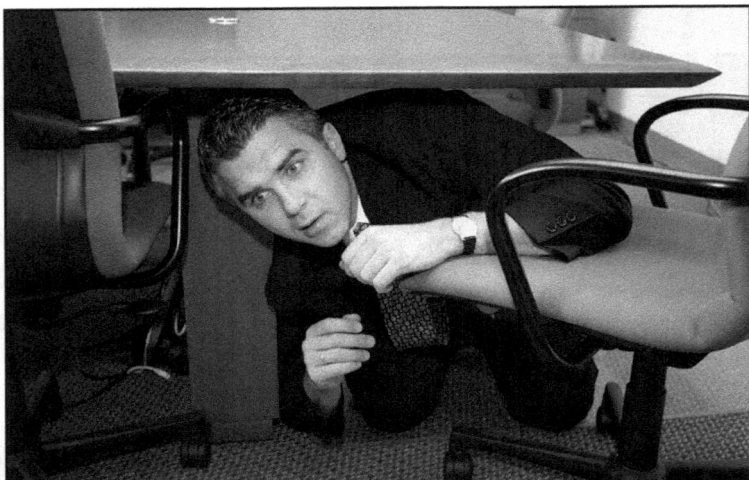

Don't forget to silence your cellphone when hiding from an active shooter.

the element of surprise. Positions of concealment include: behind doors, under desks, the dark, behind concrete walls, filing cabinets, under stairwells, large and tall objects. When hiding, remember to silence your cell phone. WARNING: Don't forget that positions of concealment are not positions of cover and do not protect you from the assailant's gun fire.

3. **Take action against the shooter.** This should only be done if your life or the life of a loved one is in immediate danger. Try to get the advantage and surprise the gunman by attacking him from behind. Try to gain immediate control of the weapon, and stay clear from the line of fire. While controlling the weapon try to attack him with head butt strikes to the nose, knee strikes to the groin and stomach, foot stomps on his toes and biting viciously into his neck, ears and face. Be relentless and don't stop until he releases hold of his weapon.

• If you are taken hostage, remain as calm as possible. Don't argue, question, or lecture your captors. Wait for a solid opportunity to escape and take it. Don't hesitate, but don't attempt escape prematurely.

• If you are taken hostage, prepare yourself for possible verbal and physical abuse, as well as lack of food, water, and sanitation.

• If ever you are unfortunate enough to be wounded by a gunshot, expect the following symptoms: Severe pain, burning sensation in the wound, breathlessness, reduced vision, potential lack of mobility, anger, fear response, and a tendency to lose your nerve.

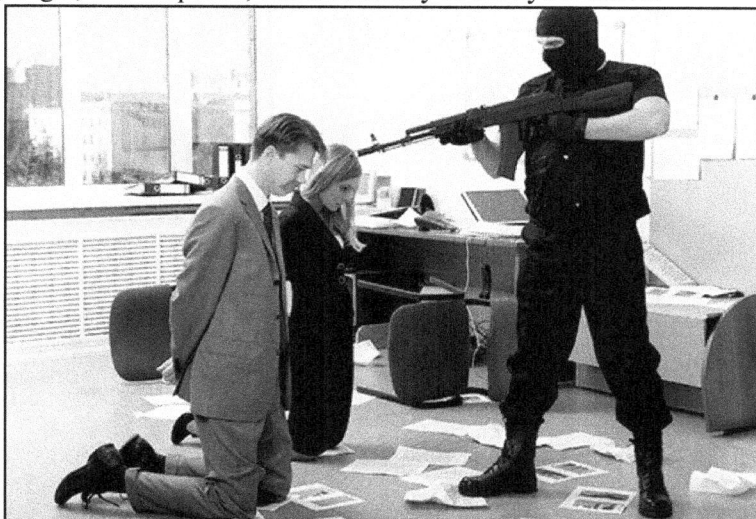

If you are taken hostage by an active shooter, remain as calm as possible. Don't argue, question, or lecture your captor.

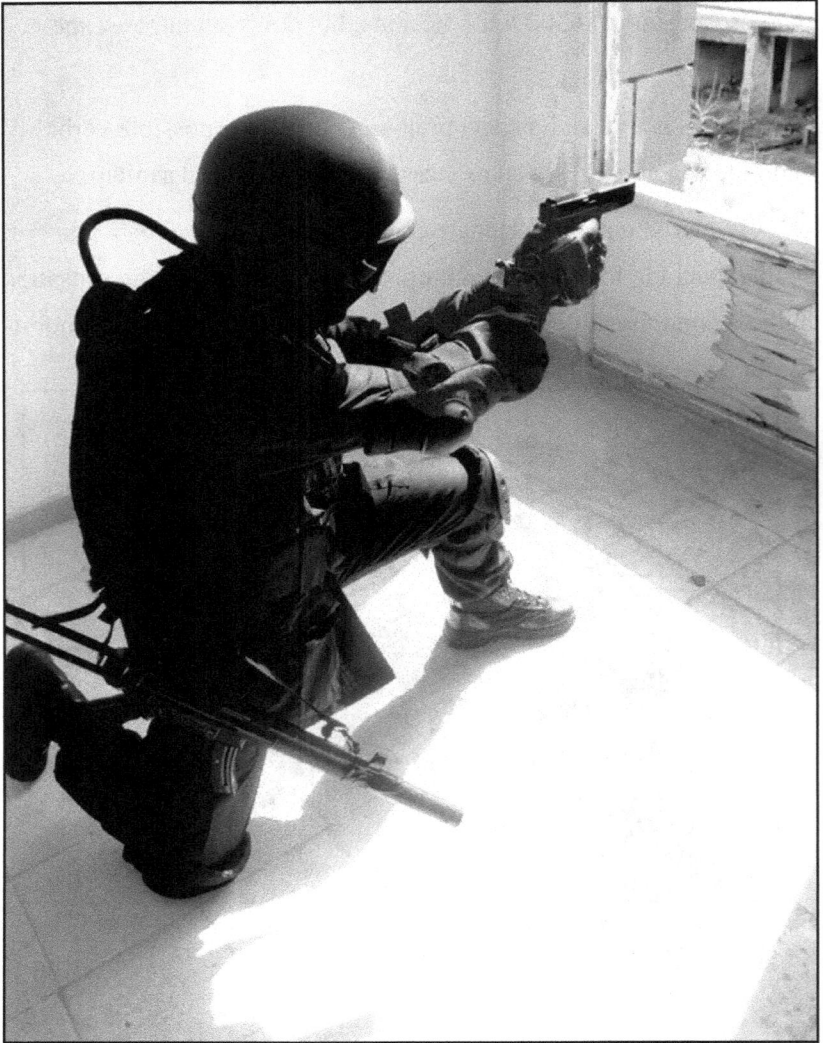

When faced with an active shooter situation, remember to keep low at all times. You don't want to be in the line of fire between the police and the gunman.

Chapter Four
Child Safety

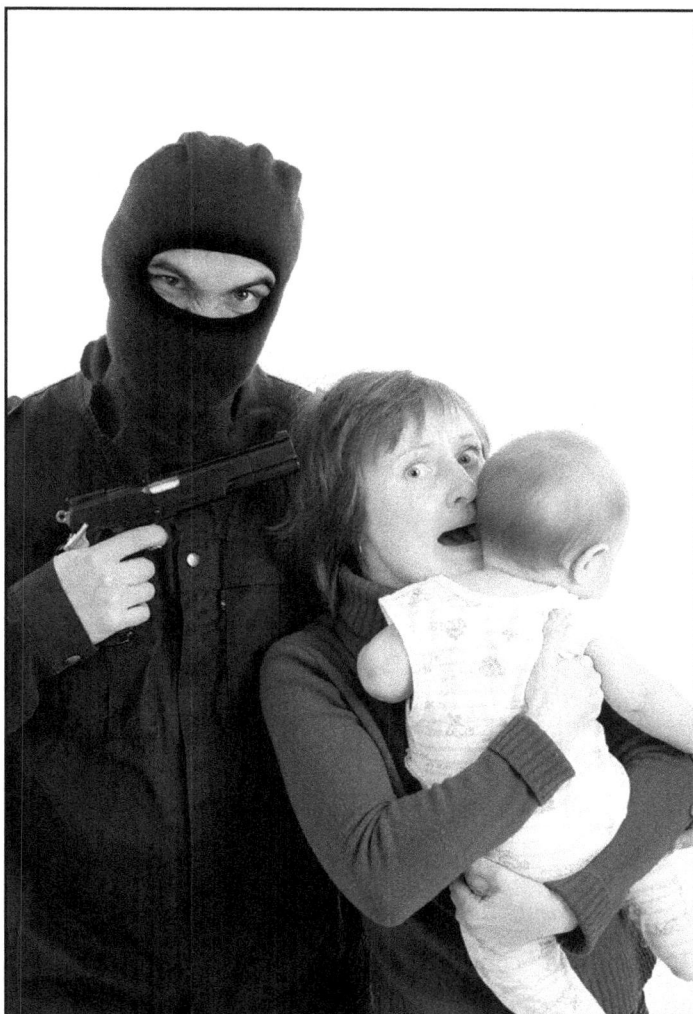

Self-Defense Tips and Tricks

- Instruct your children not to talk to strangers.

- Teach your children not to accept gifts from strangers.

- Do not allow your children to use recreational play areas unless they are supervised by responsible adults whom you know.

- When teaching street safety to your kids, emphasize caution, not fear.

- Teach your kids to routinely inform you of their whereabouts.

- Instruct your children that no one has the right to touch their bodies except the family physician.

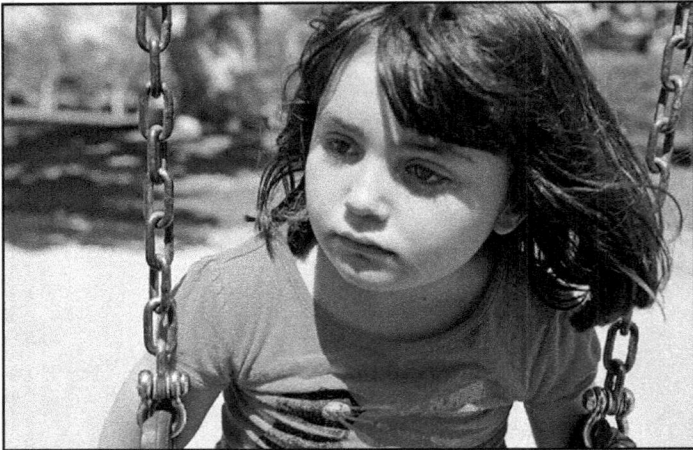

Never leave your child alone in recreational areas.

- Teach your kids how to dial 911 in case of an emergency.

- Never leave children alone in a car, not even for a few seconds.

- Don't put your child's name on their key in case they lose it.

- If your child is going door-to-door for a school project, always accompany him or her and conduct business outside.

- Consider having your children's fingerprints taken and stored safely.

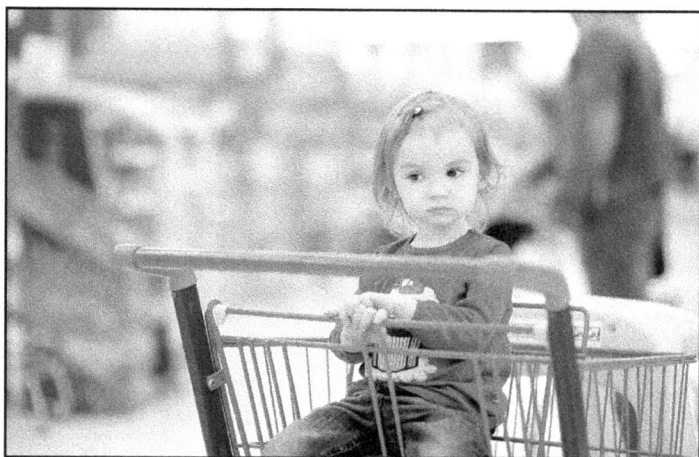

• When grocery shopping, never leave your child unattended in your cart.

• When hiring a baby-sitter, get to know the person well and always check references.

• Make it a strict rule that no company is permitted when the sitter is watching your kids.

• Consider setting up a few nanny cams in your home to keep an eye on your kids (as well as the babysitter) while you are away from them.

• Make certain your children know their names, telephone number, and address.

• Always support your kids' decisions to refuse to hug

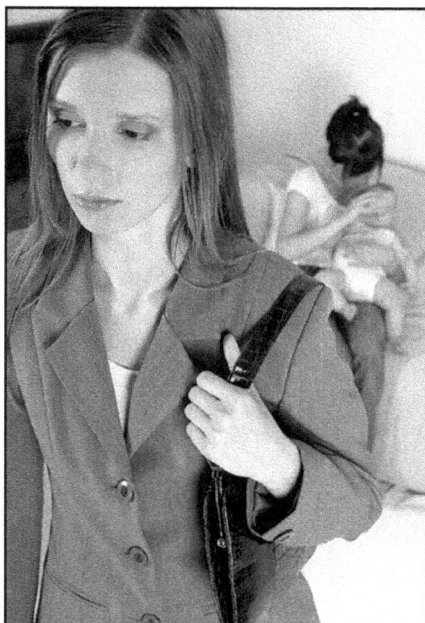

When hiring a baby-sitter, get to know the person well and always check references.

or kiss a relative like "Uncle Steve" or "Aunt Dottie." This makes it easier for them to say "No" if a stranger wants to touch them.•

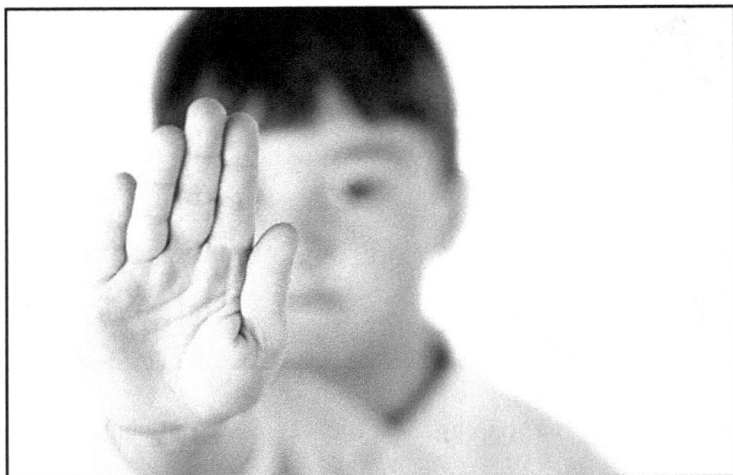

Always support your kids' decisions to refuse to hug or kiss a relative.

• Always try to accompany your children to public rest rooms. If that is not possible, then carefully monitor the length of time they are in there.

• If you suspect your child has been assaulted or sexually abused, contact the police immediately.

• For identification purposes, always have a recent photograph of your child.

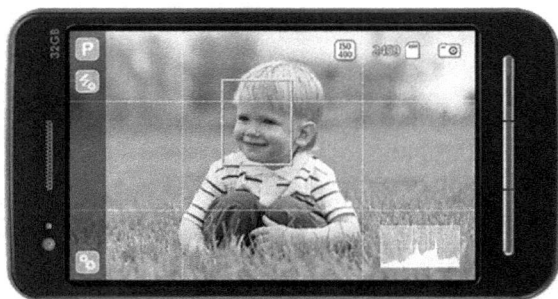

• Know where your children are at all times.

• Instruct your children not to eat candy or foodstuffs from strangers, especially on Halloween.

• Don't educate criminal predators about your children. Never write your child's name on his or her clothes, book bags, lunch box, etc.

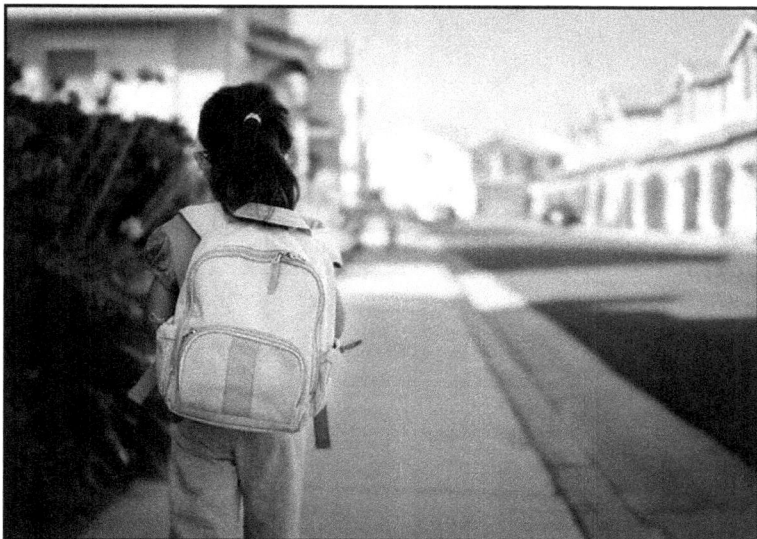

Never write your child's name on his or her clothes, book bags, lunch box, etc.

• Set up strict plan of action for picking up your kids from school, movies, or friends' homes.

• Teach your kids to come to you if they read anything on the Internet that makes them feel uneasy or uncomfortable.

• If you child own a cell phone, instruct them not to give out their number to strangers or publish it on social sites like Facebook.

• If your kids have a smart phone with GPS technology, instruct them to only use social mapping features with only close friends.

• Teach your children not to keep secrets, especially from you.

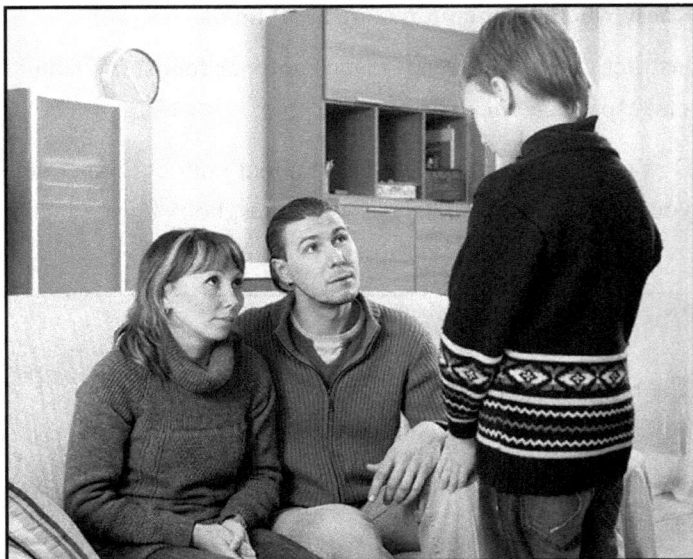

Teach your children not to keep secrets, especially from you.

• Teach your kids to talk openly with you about mistreatment or bullying. If your child is being bullied, get answers to the following important questions:

1. Who is involved?

2. What was said?

3. What happened?

4. Were there any witnesses? What did they say and do?

5. When does the bullying occur?

6. Where does it happen?

7. Was there adult supervision?

8. Are there video cameras in the area recording activities?

9. Who has been told about the bullying and what have they done?

10. How long has this been occurring?

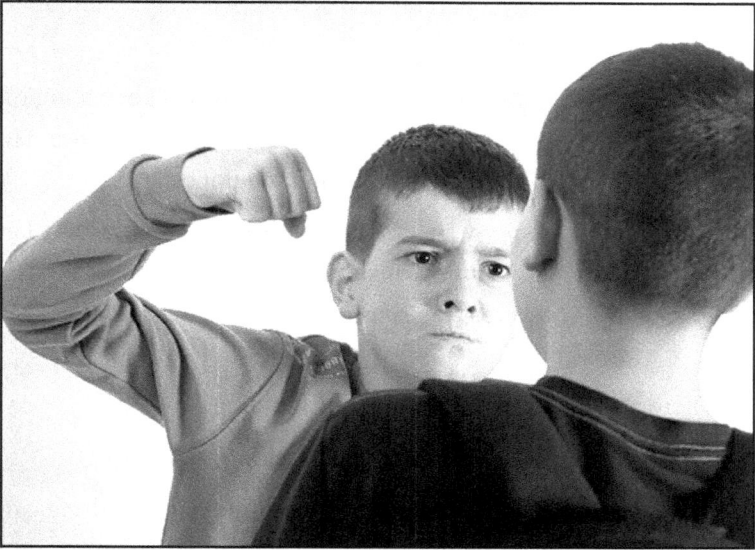

• Teach your kids to walk with confidence on the streets and in school.

• If your child is being bullied at school, remain calm and imme-

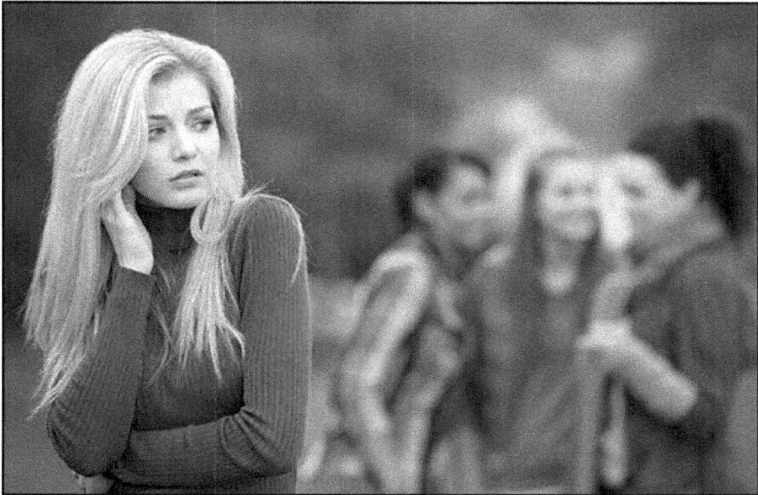

Bullying is not just limited to the physical plane. Name-calling, teasing, taunting, and insulting can be just as damaging to a person.

diately contact the bully's parents and school personnel (including the teacher and principle).

• If your child is being bullied on a regular basis, keep a log of all the events. If there are any physical signs of injury or abuse, take pictures and report them to the school and the police.

• Keep in mind, bullying is not just limited to the physical plane. Name calling, teasing, taunting, insulting, public humiliation, hazing, group exclusion, and spreading rumors can be just as damaging to a person.

• There are generally three forms of bullying:

1. **Physical** - pushing, hitting, and kicking.

2. **Verbal** - name calling, teasing, taunting, and insulting can be just as damaging to a person.

3. **Relationship** - includes group exclusion, lies and rumors, hazing, harassment, and humiliation.

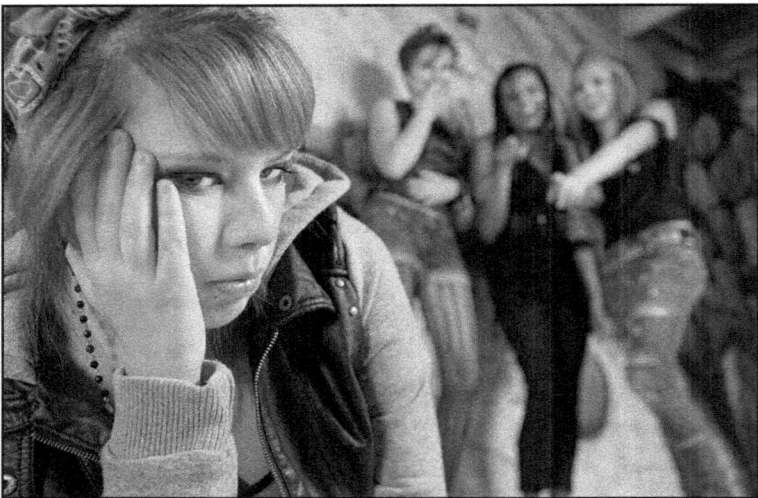

Relationship bullying includes some of the following: hazing, continual harassment, public humiliation, intentionally excluding someone from a group and spreading rumors or lies about someone.

• If you own a firearm and have children in your house, do not make guns a taboo subject. Doing so can elicit children's curiosity and possibly lead them to investigate guns on their own.

• When discussing guns with your children, be certain to answer all of their questions. If you don't know an answer to a particular question, speak with a qualified firearms instructor or a knowledgeable police officer.

If your child finds a gun in your absence, teach them the following four safety rules:

1. Stop where you are.

2. Don't touch the gun.

3. Leave immediately.

4. Tell a trustworthy adult.

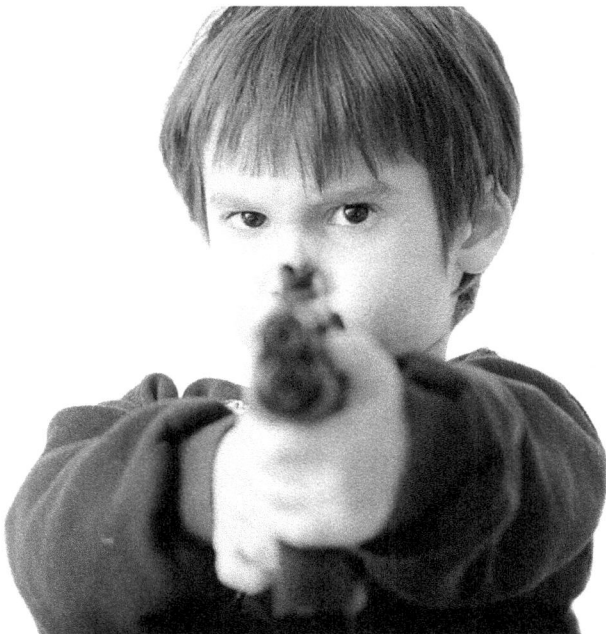

Chapter Five
Travel Safety

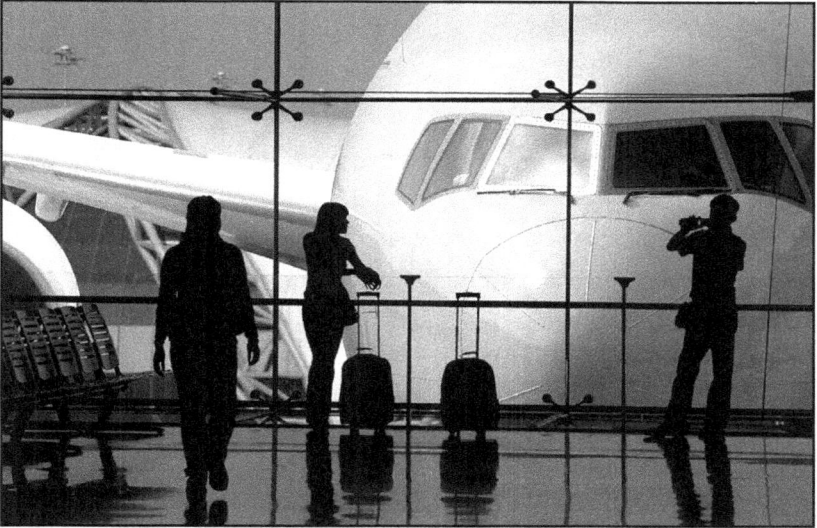

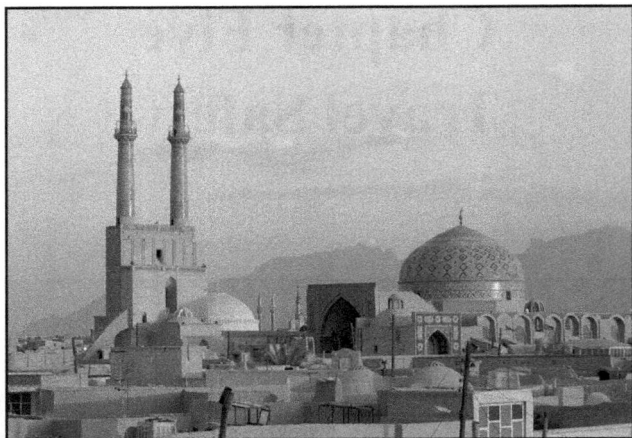

• Avoid political hot spots. Listen in advance to the news media for stories on places you plan to visit and learn about the political situation there. Even be careful of so-called stable democracies (consider the attacks that have taken place in England and Italy). No matter where your political views lie, you don't want to be an innocent victim. Call the State Department for information on countries you plan to visit.

• Avoid leaving your car in airport parking lots. Take a taxi or ask a friend for a lift.

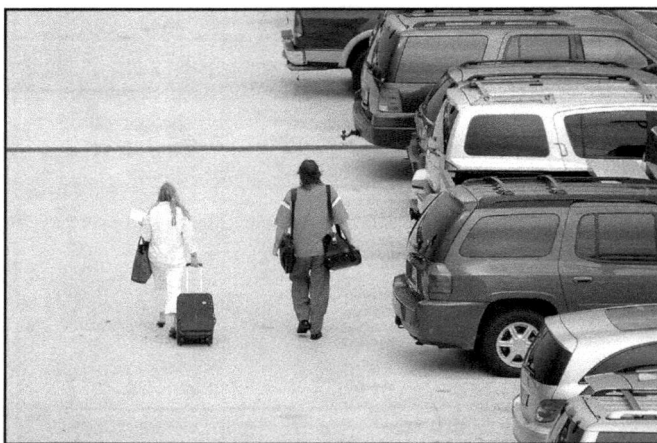

If possible, avoid leaving your car in airport parking lots.

90

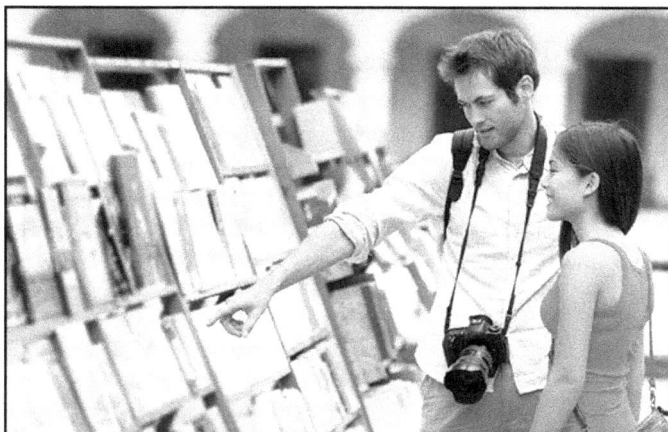

• Don't look like a tourist and wander around alone if you can avoid it.

• Try to travel light. Use hard shell luggage to avoid easy theft from soft travel bags.

• Always research (in advance) the basic information about your destination(s).

• Do not display large amounts of money when paying a bill.

• Avoid reading road maps in public places (restaurants, hotel

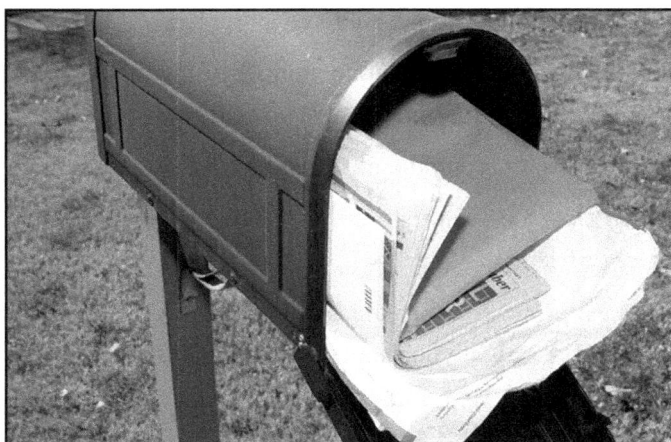

Arrange to have your mail picked up when you are away.

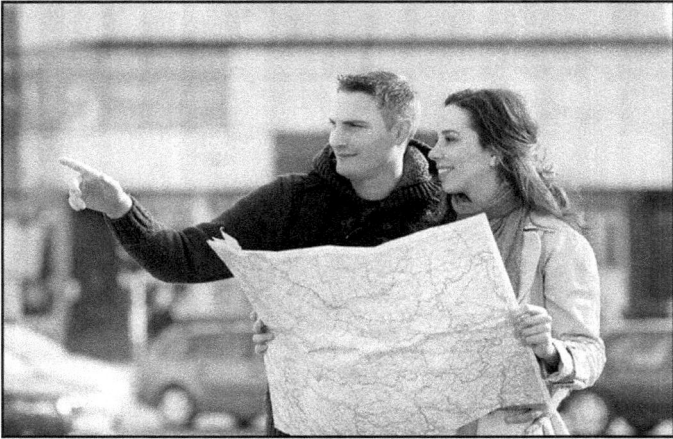

When traveling, avoid reading road maps in public places.

lobbies, gas stations, etc.) You don't want strangers to know that you are traveling.

• Before traveling, visit your physician and get all the necessary vaccinations or immunizations for the destinations you are visiting.

• When on vacation, leave a car in the driveway and have the paper and mail stopped. The post office will hold your mail.

• When away, try to have your house appear to be occupied. Install timers on lights, TVs, and radios, and change the intervals. Also ask a friend or neighbor to keep an eye on things.

• Know the location and phone number of the U.S. Embassy and consular office in any foreign country you visit.

• Plan trips with reputable travel and touring agents.

• Leave a copy of your entire travel itinerary with a trusted family member or friend.

• The best protection for your home when traveling is to have a friend or relative stay at your house while you are gone.

• When traveling, don't tell strangers you are traveling alone.

• Never leave your belongings unattended in public spaces.

• Avoid aisle seats on planes. They put you right next to where hijackers will be moving up and down the plane and possibly choosing hostages or victims. Instead, request window, exit, or rear seats.

• If your plane is hijacked, remain calm and alert, keep your mouth shut, don't draw attention to yourself, and never volunteer to do anything. Above all, don't debate political or other issues. If your captors demand identification, surrender your passport immediately.

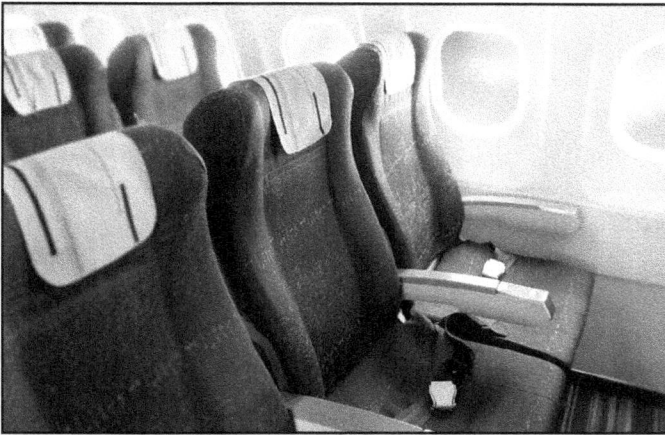

If possible, avoid aisle seats on planes.

• If you are on a hijacked plane that is stormed by a rescue team, dive for cover, stay down, and don't move until told to do so. If you must move, belly crawl while staying low to the ground.

• When traveling abroad, avoid wearing ethnic or religious clothing. Try to blend with the local population and don't wear T-shirts or clothing sporting political slogans.

• If you work for the government, don't bring official documents on board the plane. Pack them away. You don't want to be identified as an agent of the government. If you travel on a diplomatic passport, your agency will brief you accordingly.

• Try to book direct, secure-route flights to foreign countries. Stopover flights increase the likelihood of bomb emplacement or

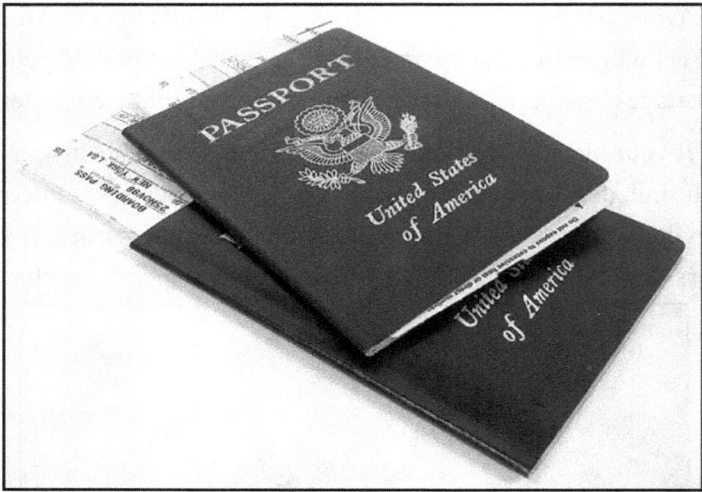

other terrorist activity.

• When sightseeing, carry a copy of your passport's data, keep your actual passport locked in your hotel safe.

• Your passport is not a "get out of jail" card. Keep in mind that if you break local laws while abroad, your U.S. passport won't help you avoid arrest or possible prosecution.

• Make all reservations at reputable hotels. Be familiar with

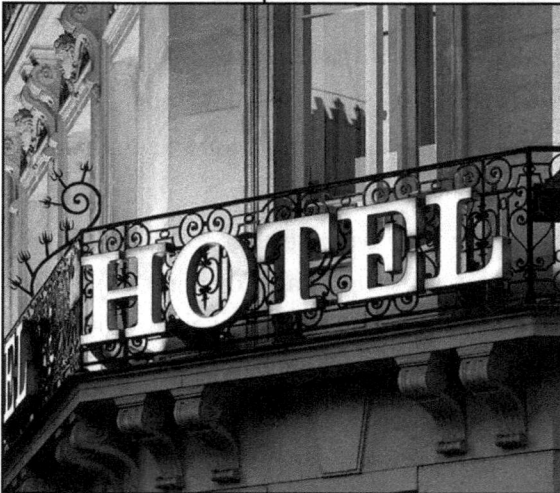

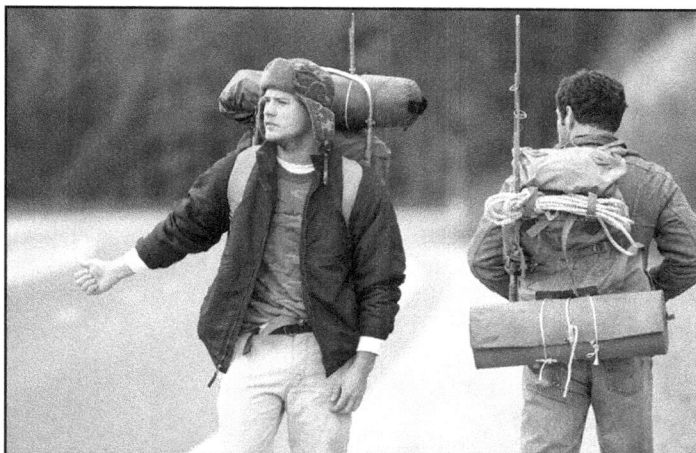

Hitchhiking is dangerous, especially in foreign countries.

exits, entrances, rest rooms, and telephones.

• Avoid hitchhiking, especially in foreign countries.

• To prevent being taken by surprise, get into the habit of looking back when you get up to leave somewhere.

Before traveling, find out what medical services your health insurance will cover when you are overseas. If your current insur-

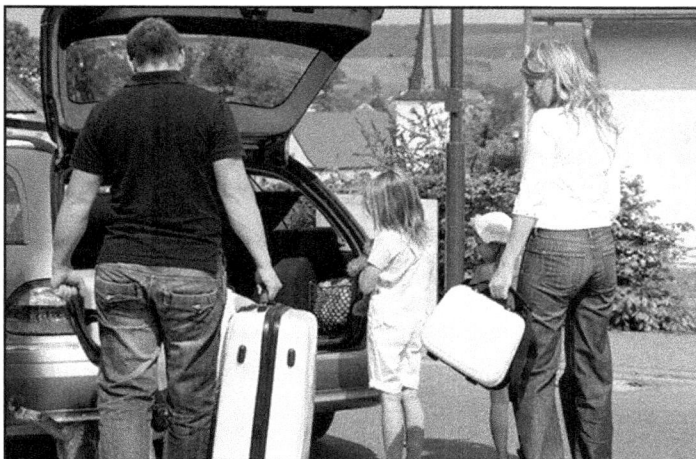

Avoid packing your car in public. If possible, do it privately in your garage.

ance policy does not cover you when abroad, consider purchasing a short-term policy that will.

• Some countries have strict restrictions on prescription medications. To prevent any hassles when traveling, consider getting a letter

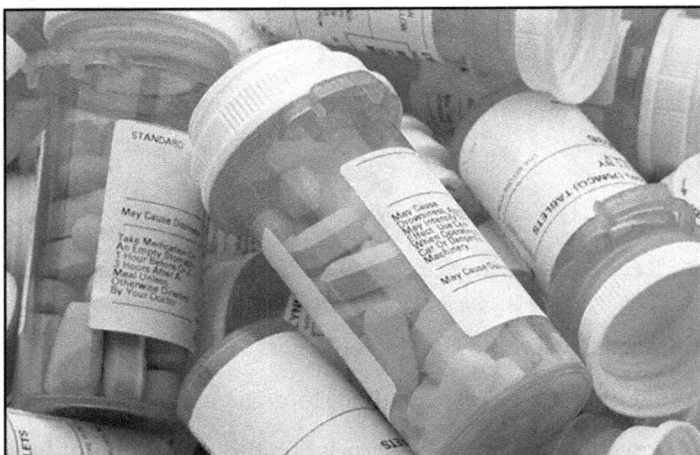

from your physician in case you are questioned about it.

• As soon as you arrive in another country, go to the authorities and try to find out where the dangerous areas are. Every city has them, and the police know where they are.

• Vary your travel routes and times, and always maintain a low profile.

• Never give money to strangers or beggars on the street.

• Don't let the public know that you are leaving on a trip. Avoid packing your car in public. If possible, do it privately in your garage.

• If you are traveling by automobile, avoid loading up your car the night before you leave. Remember, a fully packed car tells potential burglars that you will be away.

• When in the airport, report any suspicious people or activities to security personnel.

• If you are traveling with your kids, inform them not to make jokes or false threats about security issues.

• Make certain you understand the exchange rate before you travel.

• Before traveling, find out whether your cell phone has roaming capabilities at your destination. If not, consider, renting a phone once you arrive.

• When you are away, ask a trustworthy neighbor to use your trash can and take it out at the curb and bring it back on trash day.

• Ask your neighbor to park their car in your driveway while you are gone.

• Never announce your vacation plans or post pictures of your trip on social media sites like Facebook. Burglars have been known to use social media sites to determine if homeowners are away.

• Before you take your trip overseas, photograph or scan your

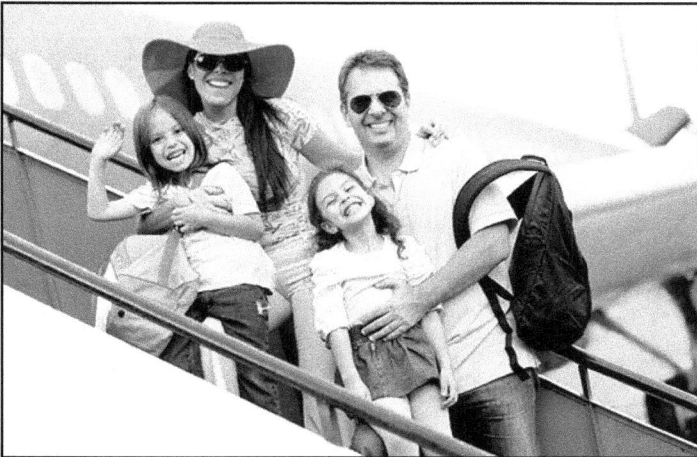

Never post pictures of your trip on social media sites like Facebook.

travel documents and email them to yourself. - that way your papers won't go missing even if your bags do.

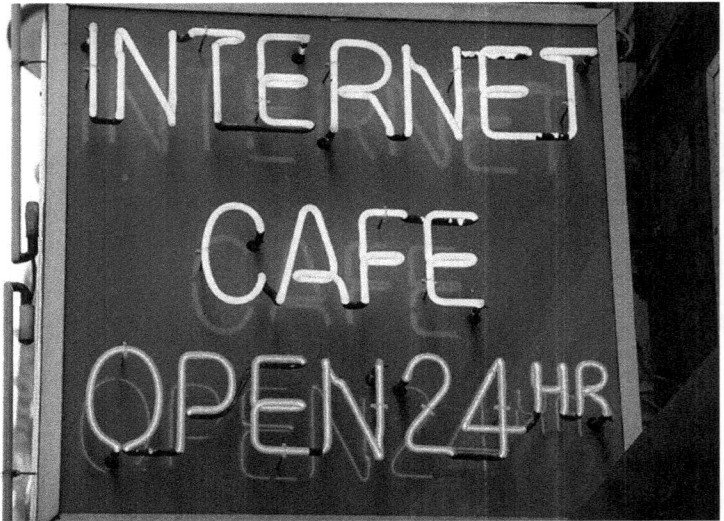

When traveling, avoid using your credit card at an Internet cafe.

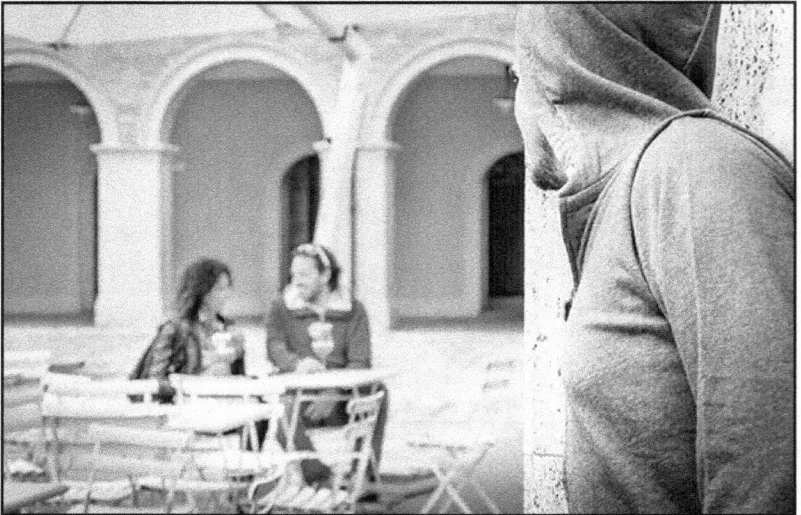

When on vacation, remain alert of your surroundings. You never know who might be watching you.

• Be very careful who you pick as a travel companion. The wrong person can compromise your safety and put you at risk. If they are doing something that is dangerous, tell them immediately. If they continue to be conduct themselves in an unsafe manner, consider parting ways.

• When you arrive at your hotel for the first time, make a mental not of all the fire escapes on your floor.

• While it might be tempting to check your email while away, avoid using your credit card at an Internet cafe.

• When checking in, always keep a close eye on your luggage, purse, etc. This is especially important if the hotel lobby is very busy.

• When making a hotel reservation, avoid being gender specific. Always use your first initial and your last name.

• If you are a woman and traveling alone, request that your room

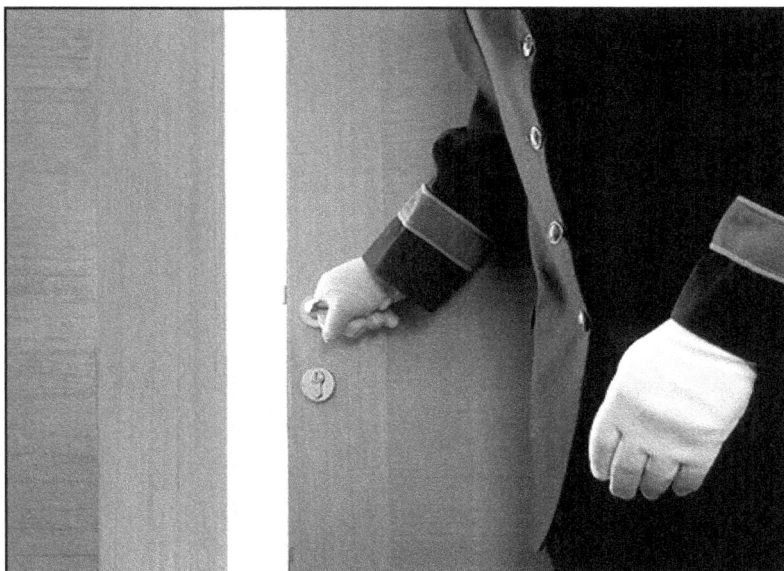

If you are a woman and traveling alone, request that your room service order be delivered by a female.

service order be delivered by a female.

• Avoid booking hotel rooms that are in isolated areas of the building. Specifically request a room in heavily trafficked areas.

• Do not accept a guest room on the first floor. They are generally the easiest to break into.

• Discreetly request to the hotel clerk not to announce your room number. Instead, ask him to write it down for you.

• Make certain your guest room has a working smoke detector.

• Whenever you are in your guest room, always leave the "do not disturb" sign on the door.

• To maximize your safety in case of a fire, do not book a room

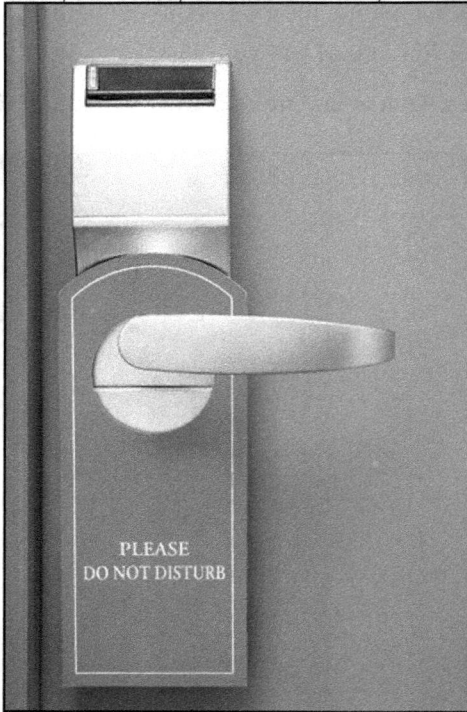

When you arrive at your guest room, always inspect the door and lock and make certain it's functioning properly.

above the 6th floor. Fire department ladders can't only reach past the 6th floor.

• Never stay in a guest room that does not have a working telephone.

• Don't accept a guest room that is directly connected to another suite. Insist on another room.

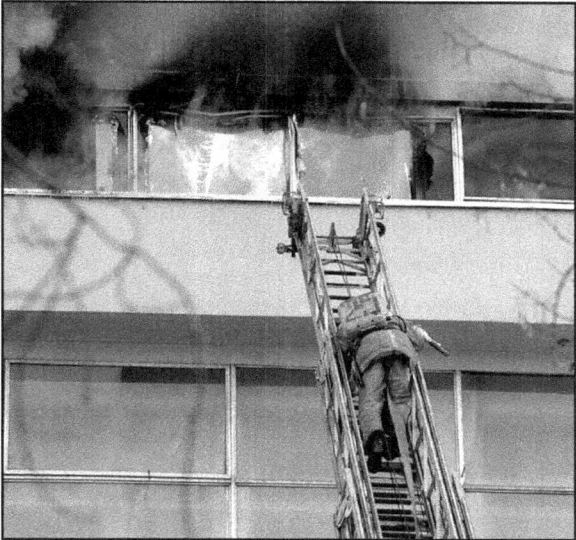

• If and when you leave your hotel room, leave the television on. This will help discourage criminals from breaking into your guest room.

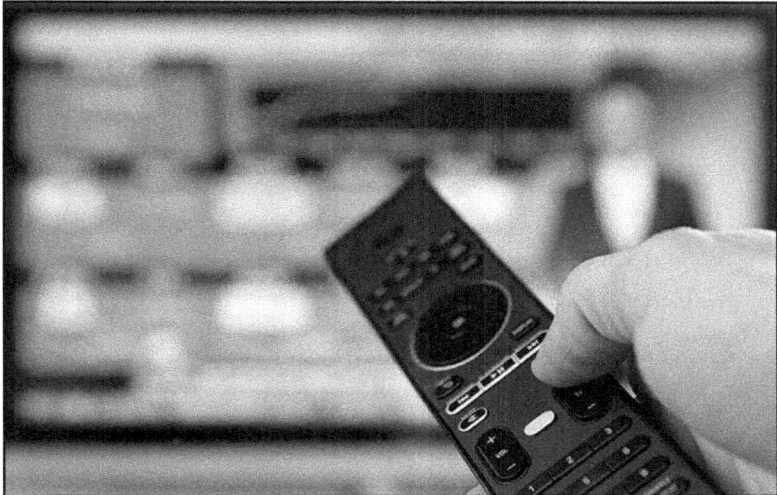

• Always have your key in hand as your approach your room. Be quick and efficient. Avoid lingering in the hallways and corridors of your hotel.

• If you must carry valuables with you while traveling, always keep them hidden in your guest room. Better yet, store them in the hotel safe.

• When traveling abroad, do not take photographs of the locals. This is especially important when it comes to military personnel, police, and military installations. In some countries, you can get arrested and convicted for espionage.

• Learn the words for "no", "police" and "help" in the language of the country you are visiting. They will can come in handy.

• As tempting as it might be, don't haggle or talk with street vendors. If they approach you, say "no" and quickly move on your way.

• Try to avoid wandering alone in a foreign country. Stick with tour groups.

• Never ask strangers for directions (including the locals), instead ask someone who serves in an official capacity.

• Always dress modestly. Avoid provocative or sexy attire. You never want to bring attention to yourself or your partner. Remember,

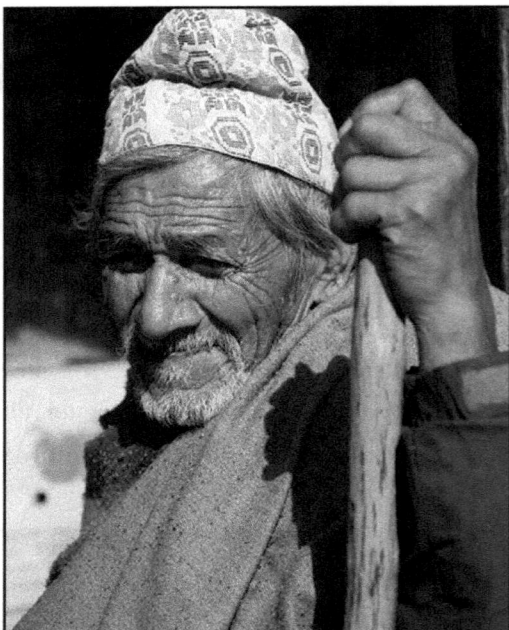

the goal is to blend in with everyone else.

• Before visiting a foreign country, be knowledgeable of the culture and its customs. Remember, to be respectful!

• Leave expensive jewelry and watches at home.

• Avoid disclosing information about your vacation to taxi drivers.

• If you are going away for an extended period of time, arrange to have someone cut the lawn.

• If you have the option, try to arrive at your destination during the daylight hours.

Self-Defense Tips and Tricks

Chapter Six
Fighting Back Tips

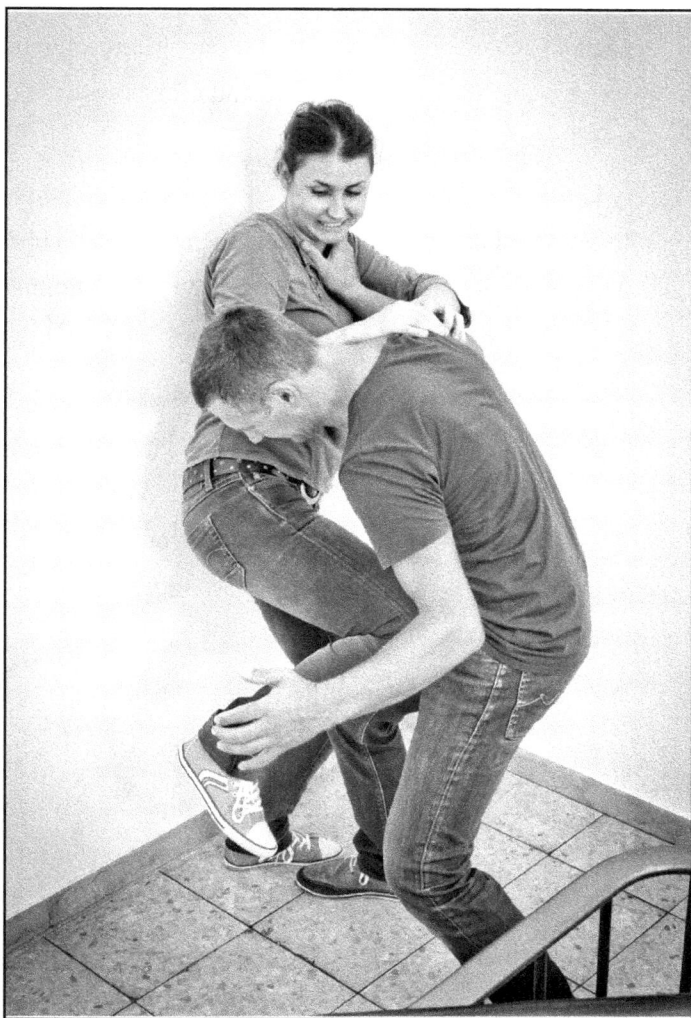

Self-Defense Tips and Tricks

- Always keep your eyes opened and focused on your adversary when fighting.

- Always exhale when executing a self-defense technique.

- Breathing is one of the most important and often neglected aspects of self-defense. Proper breathing promotes muscular relaxation and increases the speed and efficiency of your self-defense techniques.

- Try to avoid fearful blinking when attacked. Remember, a split second link could leave you vulnerable. While blinking is a natural reflex, it can be reduced or possibly eliminated when fighting.

- Avoid tensing your muscles when executing your self-defense technique. Remember, muscular relaxation promotes speed.

- Try to maintain a 45° angle stance from your adversary when fighting. This will reduce target opportunities for the adversary and maximize your ability to fight back.

- Always aim through your target when punching.

- Always execute a strike with maximum speed.

- If you decide to fight back against a criminal, always do so with 100% commitment. Anything less can get you seriously injured or possibly killed.

- Always assume your adversary has a weapon and is capable of using it.

- Remember to torque hips and upper body in the same direction as your striking limb. This maximizes the power.

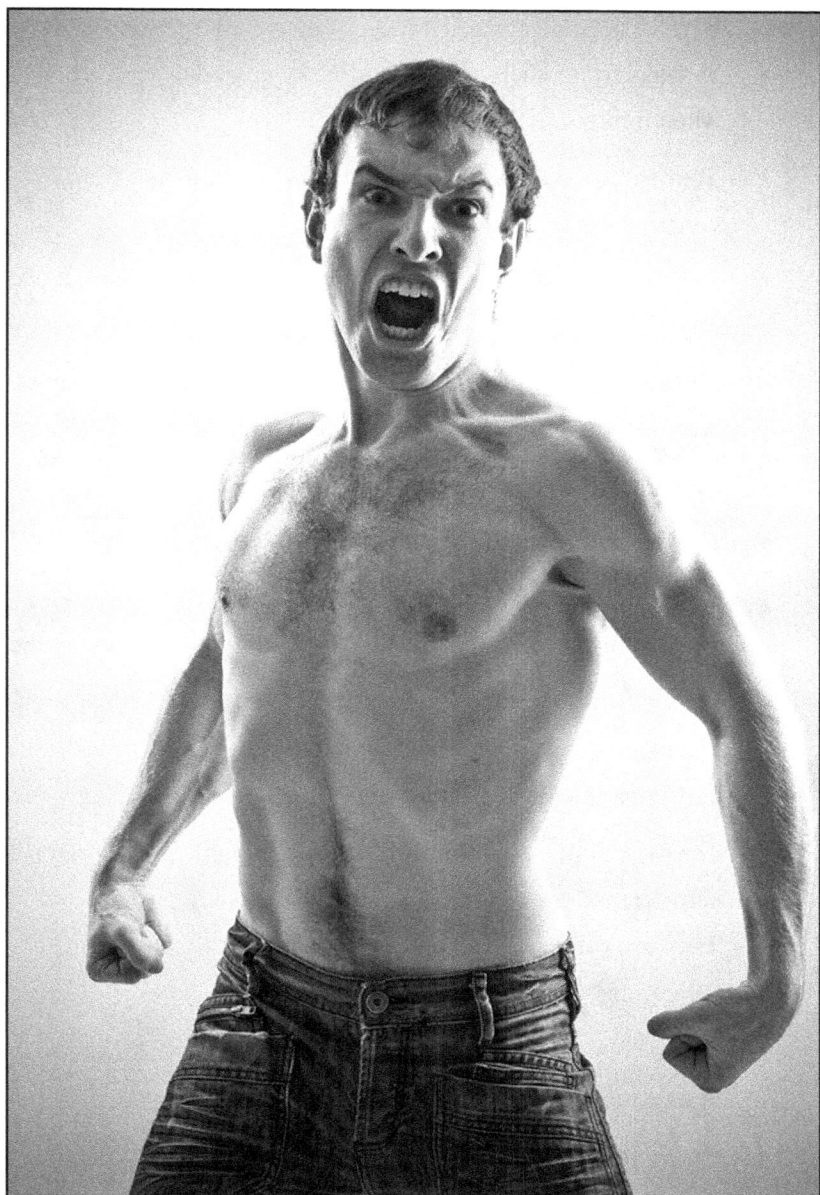

107

Self-Defense Tips and Tricks

- Remember to keep your wrists straight when delivering punching techniques.

- Always try to keep your chin slightly angled downward when fighting.

- Remember to deploy your closest body weapon to the adversary's closest target.

- Remember to keep your hands up when fighting your adversary.

- Always approach self-defense in a simple and direct manner. Avoid flashy or complex techniques and maneuvers.

- Learn to trust your instincts. They are usually right!

- Always have a strategic purpose behind every move you make in the streets.

- Believe in yourself, despite how bad things might look at the moment.

- If danger is imminent, strike first, strike fast, and strike with authority and keep the pressure on!

- Try to minimize kicking techniques in a fight. For real-world self-defense applications, hand techniques are preferred. They are safer and generally more efficient than kicking techniques.

- If you are involved in a self-defense altercation, always be cognizant and leery of spectators.

- Remember to follow through with your striking techniques. Target penetration leads to incapacitation!

Self-Defense Tips and Tricks

- Remember to keep your wrists straight when delivering punching techniques.

- Always try to keep your chin slightly angled downward when fighting.

- Remember to deploy your closest body weapon to the adversary's closest target.

- Remember to keep your hands up when fighting your adversary.

- Always approach self-defense in a simple and direct manner. Avoid flashy or complex techniques and maneuvers.

- Learn to trust your instincts. They are usually right!

- Always have a strategic purpose behind every move you make in the streets.

- Believe in yourself, despite how bad things might look at the moment.

- If danger is imminent, strike first, strike fast, and strike with authority and keep the pressure on!

- Try to minimize kicking techniques in a fight. For real-world self-defense applications, hand techniques are preferred. They are safer and generally more efficient than kicking techniques.

- If you are involved in a self-defense altercation, always be cognizant and leery of spectators.

- Remember to follow through with your striking techniques. Target penetration leads to incapacitation!

108

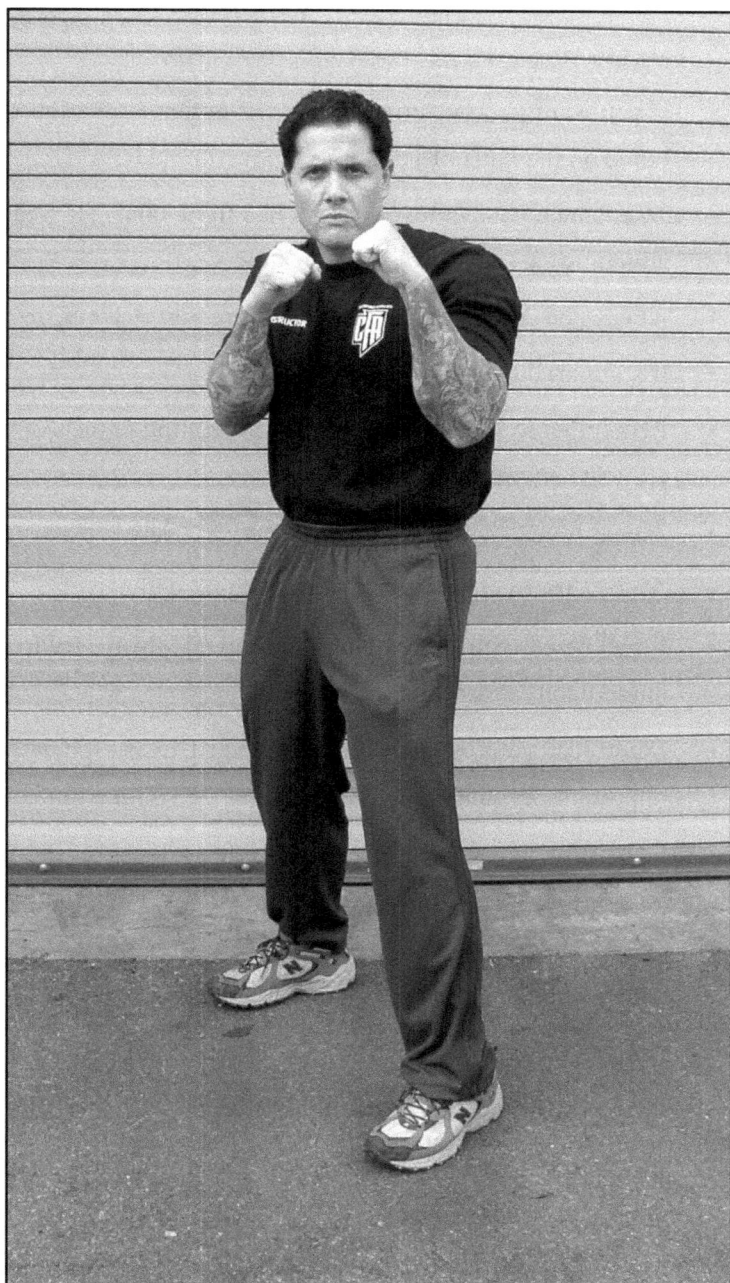

Self-Defense Tips and Tricks

- Avoid distractions and always stay focused on your immediate threat.

- If you want to move quickly in a self-defense situation, try to move on the balls of your feet.

- To enhance your footwork skills in a fight, consider wearing athletic shoes when walking the streets.

- Always be certain of your target before you strike it.

- It's important to stay relaxed under stress.

- Remember to move cautiously when fighting in dark or crowded environments.

- Never forget that your mind is your greatest weapon.

- Always try to make your adversary think defensively.

- When faced with a threatening individual, always try to immediately determine his intent.

- Never lose your balance when fighting. This is especially important if you are unarmed and attacked with a knife.

- Learn how to execute various self-defense techniques from a variety of stances, postures, and positions. For example, practice defensive moves while you are sitting in a chair, while sunbathing, or lying in your bed.

- Learn how to move and strike simultaneously.

- Learn how to defend yourself in the dark.

- Learn how to identify which self-defense situations warrant the use of deadly force.

- Learn the appropriate counter moves to various grabs, locks,

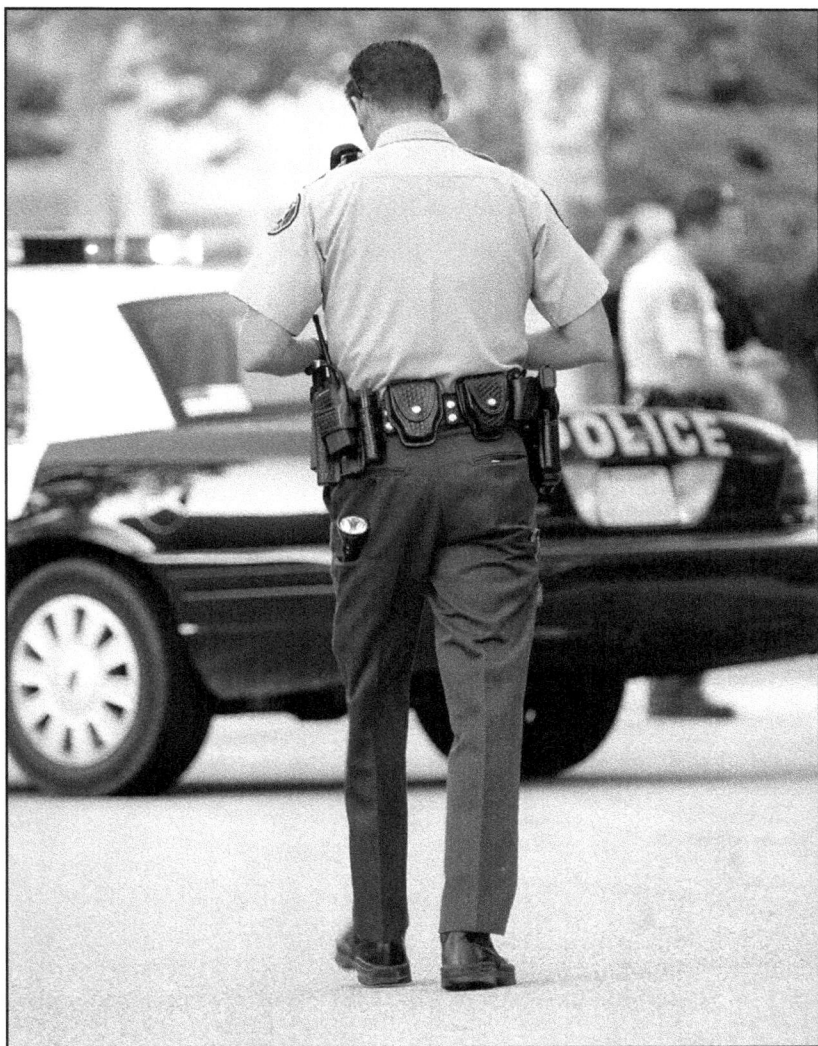

and chokes.

- Strive to make your self-defense techniques natural and instinctive. This means lots of practice and repetition. As the saying goes, "repetition is the mother of skill."

- Learn how to control your fears of violence.

- Learn how to fight from the ground..

- Learn how to recognize telegraphic movement from your adversary.

- Learn how to strike a moving target.

- Learn the medical implications behind every self-defense technique in your arsenal.

- Learn the possible reaction dynamics to every possible strike you can deliver.

- Don't make mistakes.

- Learn to scan your immediate environment for possible makeshift weapons. These are everyday objects that can be converted into offensive and defensive weapons.

- Don't smoke.

- Never show fear to your adversary.

- Never let your emotions surface when fighting. Try to be emotionless and tactical.

- To develop powerful punches, hit the heavy bag on a regular basis.

- Never strike your adversary unless it is justified in the eyes of the law.

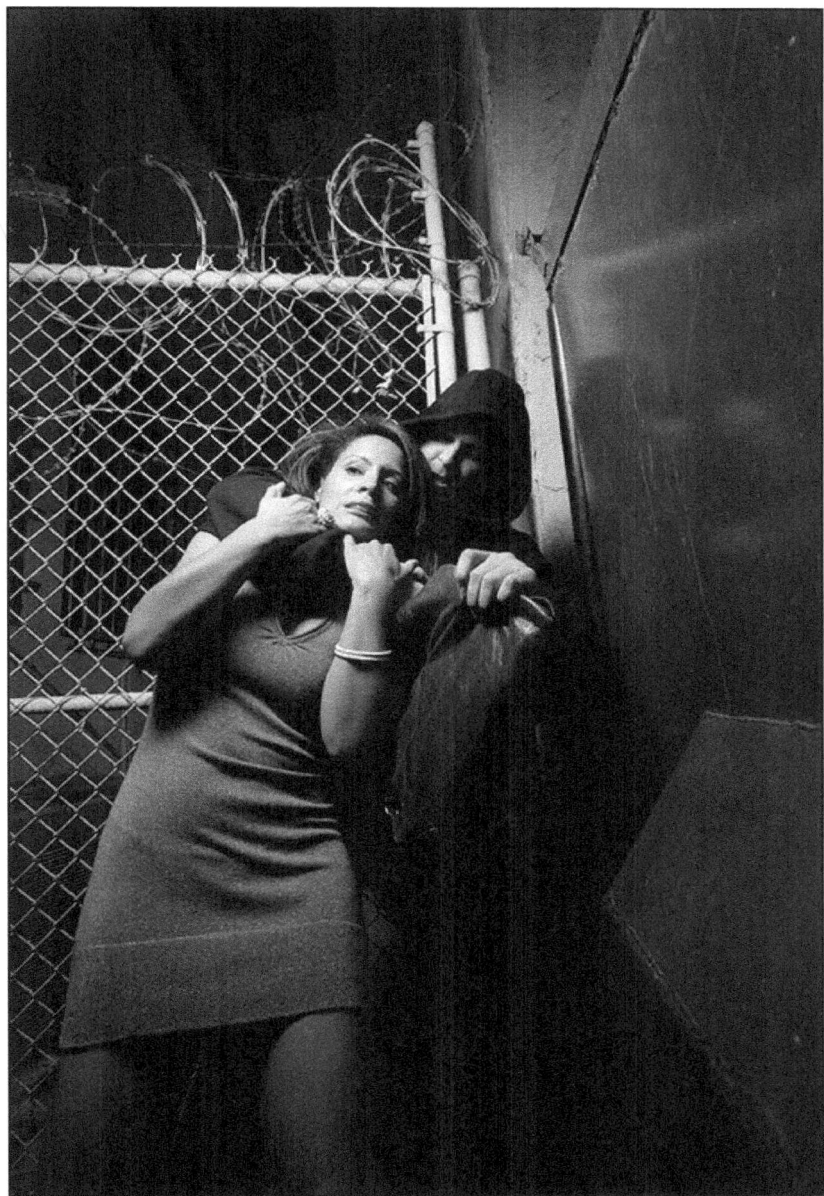

Self-Defense Tips and Tricks

- Never underestimate anyone. This includes teenagers and seniors.

- Never perform a self-defense technique unless you are certain it will land.

- Never let your adversary get the advantage of the first strike.

- Never turn your back to your adversary.

- Never threaten anyone. If you have to fight - then fight.

- Never cock your arm back prior to striking your adversary. Such forms of telegraphing will get you hurt in the fight.

- Don't let your ego control your self defense arsenal.

- Don't let your assailant back you into a wall.

- When fighting back against your attacker, constantly scan your immediate surroundings for escape routes. Escape routes are various avenues or exits you can use to escape from a threatening situation.

- Remember, there is nothing cowardly about running away from a dangerous situation.

- Never get into a shoving match with your adversary. It's juvenile and robs you of your tactical advantage in a fight.

- Never telegraph your intentions.

- Don't rely on anyone to help you in a fight.

- Don't stare into your assailant's eyes. When fighting, the eyes do not provide any vital data and they can often "psych you out."

- Don't let anyone intimidate you.

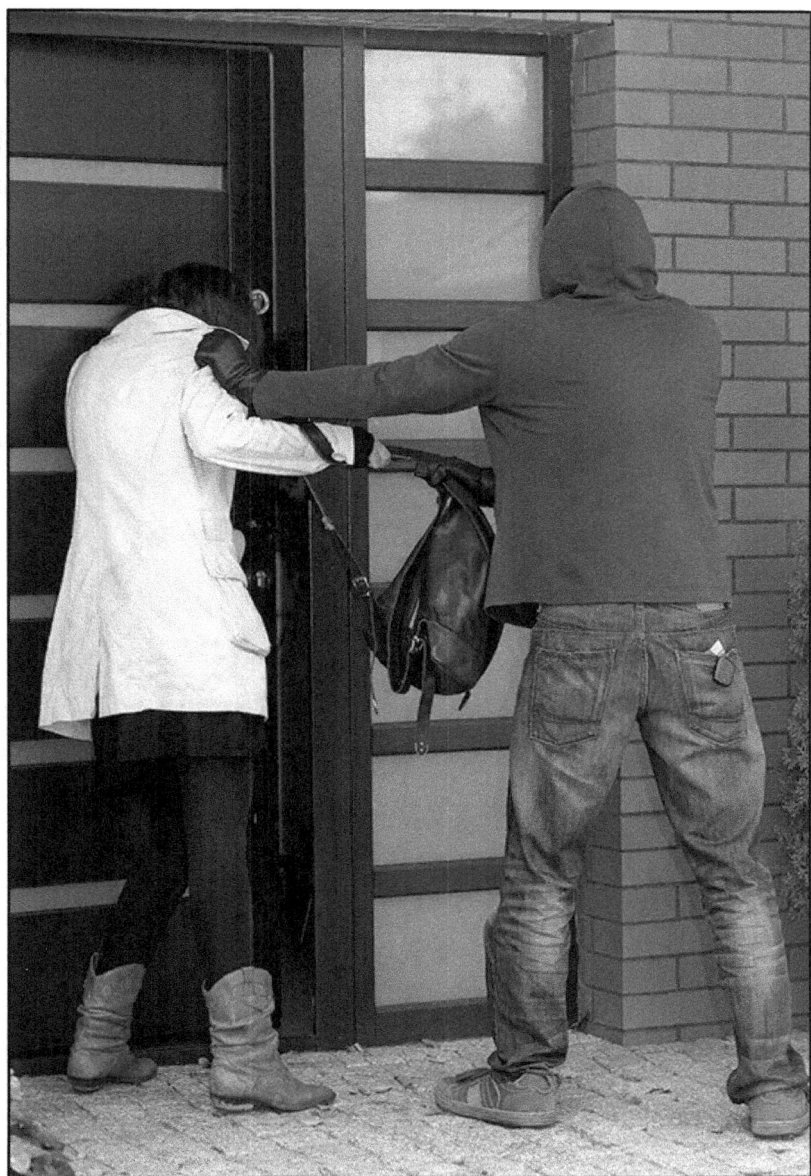

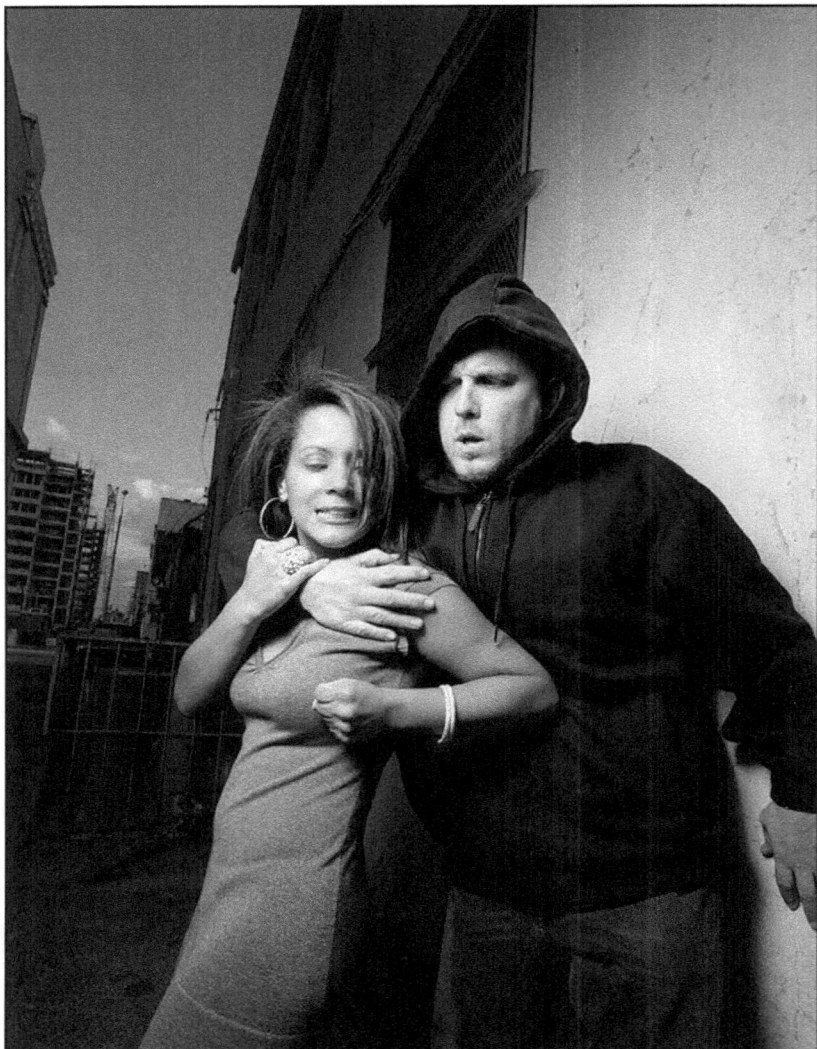

- Learn the difference between "perceptual danger" and "reasonable danger."

- Don't let multiple assailants around you. Constantly move around and look for the nearest escape route.

- Evaluate your past responses to dangerous or threatening situations. How did you do?

- Understand and accept the physiological responses to the fight or flight response.

- If you own a firearm, you have a personal responsibility to visit the gun range on a regular basis. Regular training also applies if you rely on pepper spray, stun guns or any other personal protection weapon.

- When training, regularly practice assault scenarios with fully padded assailants. A good reality-based self-defense instructor can help you with this.

- When training, you must integrate the frightening and spontaneous elements of violence safely into your routine.

- Inadequate or unrealistic self-defense training is extremely dangerous. Always train for the reality of self-defense.

- Try to work out in different environments, such as between two parked cars, and a swimming pool, on a flight of stairs, or sitting behind the wheel of your car.

- Learn to pseudospeciate your adversary. Pseudospeciation is the ability to assign inferior and sub human qualities to another criminal immediately in a threatening encounter. This psychological frame of mind is important in self-defense because it allows you to attack the assailant with vicious intent and determination. More importantly, it permits you to unleash your killer instinct immediately, while freeing you from the inherent dangers of apprehension.

- If you want to neutralize a criminal adversary, you'll need to do more than execute a single punch or strike. The truth is, most unarmed self-defense situations will require that you initiate a compound attack against your attacker. A compound attack is the logical sequence of two or more techniques strategically thrown in succession the objective is to take the fight out of the attacker and the attacker out of the fight by overwhelming his defenses with a flurry of full speed, full force strikes.

- When studying self-defense, make certain you learn how to disarm a gun as well as a knife.

- When fighting for your life, learn to tap into your killer instinct. Essentially, the killer instinct is a reservoir of energy and strength that fuels your determination to fight to the death.

- Consider learning how to use a walking stick or cane as a self-defense weapon. They appear innocuous but are extremely effective self-defense tools.

- Self-defense techniques are not enough. You must know where to strike your attacker. A criminal's anatomical targets are located in one of three possible target zones. Zone one is the head region, and it consists of targets related to his senses, including the eyes, temples, nose, chin, and back of

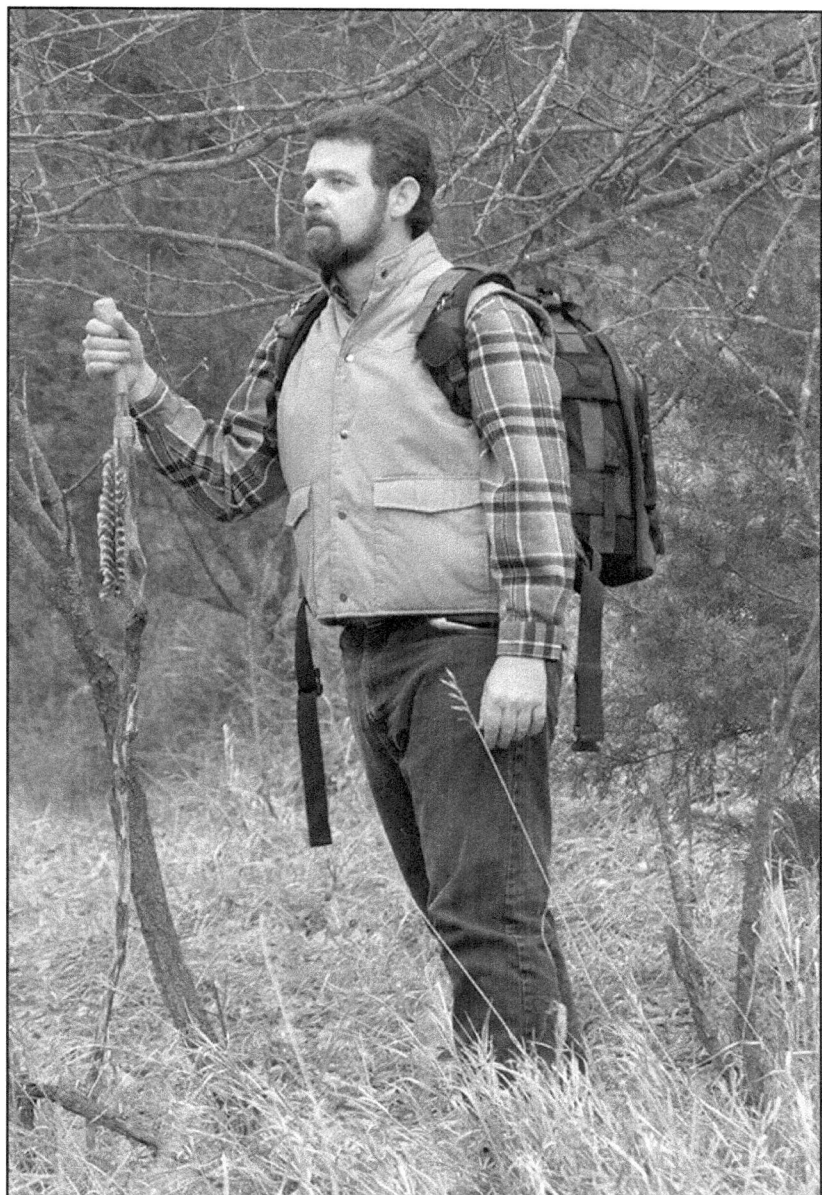

the neck. Zone two is the neck, torso, and groin region and it consists of targets related to the assailant's breathing including the throat, solar plexus, ribs, and groin. Zone three are the legs and feet and they consist of targets related to the assailants mobility, including the thighs, knees, shins, and toes.

- When defending yourself against an attack, always try to maintain a 50% weight distribution. This will provide you with the ability to move in any direction quickly and efficiently while also supplying you with the necessary stability to withstand and defend against blows and strikes.

- When assuming any type of protective stance, the distance between your feet is a critical factor. If your feet are too close to each other you will lack the necessary balance to maintain an effective fighting posture. Likewise, if your feet are too far apart you'll be too rigid and static, thus restricting your ability to move quickly. The best solution is to keep your feet approximately shoulder width apart. This will provide you with sufficient balance and stability without sacrificing mobility.

- While there are many vital targets that you need to protect when defending yourself, the most important one is your head. Your head is the computer center that controls the functioning of your entire body. Since most of your vital senses (smell, sight, hearing, and equilibrium) are stored in the head, you must keep it out of harm's way. Assuming the proper fighting stance accomplishes this.

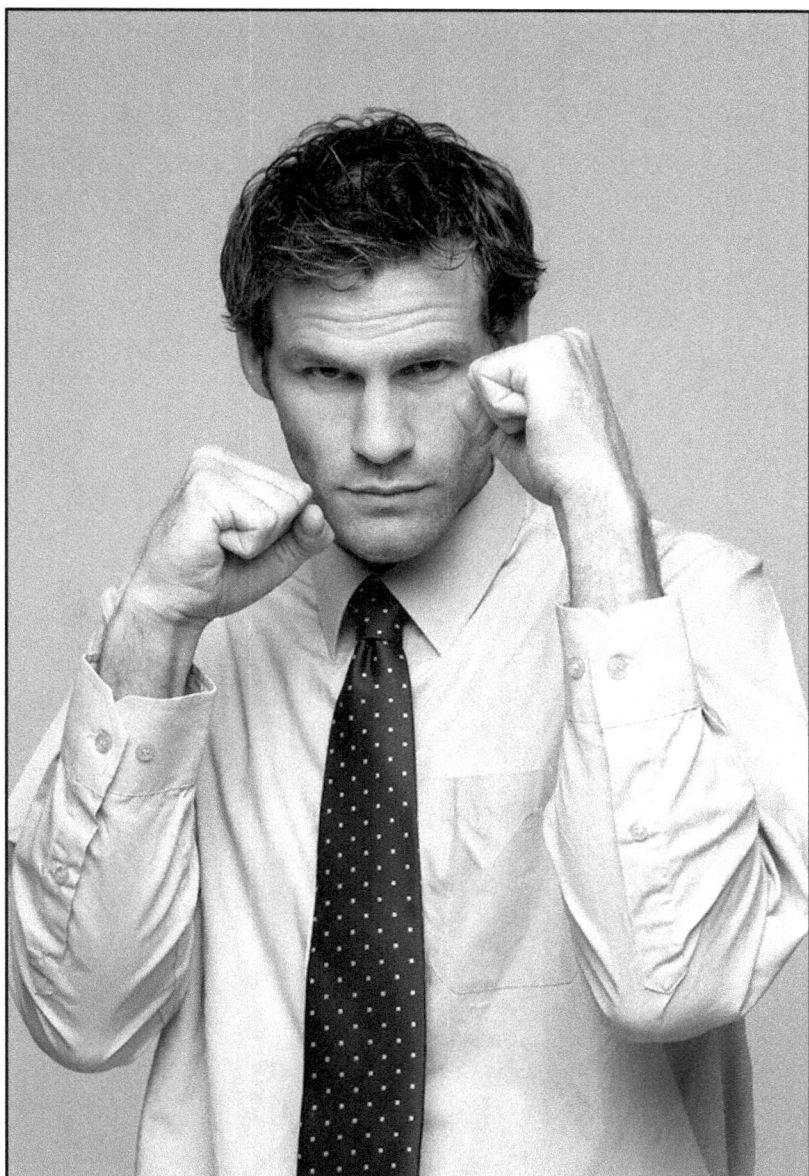

Self-Defense Tips and Tricks

Glossary of Terms

The following terms are defined in the context of Contemporary Fighting Arts and its related concepts. In many instances, the definitions bear little resemblance to those found in a standard dictionary.

A

Accuracy - The precise or exact projection of force. Accuracy is also defined as the ability to execute a combative movement with precision and exactness.

Active shooter - an individual actively engaged in killing or attempting to kill people in a confined and populated area, typically through the use of firearms.

Adaptability - The ability to physically and psychologically adjust to new or different conditions or circumstances of combat.

Aerobic Exercise - "With air." Exercise that elevates the heart rate to a training level for a prolonged period of time, usually 30 minutes.

Agility - An attribute of combat. One's ability to move his or her body quickly and gracefully.

Ambidextrous - The ability to perform with equal facility on both the right and left sides of the body.

Attributes of Combat - The physical, mental, and spiritual qualities that enhance combat skills and tactics.

B

Balance - One's ability to maintain equilibrium while stationary or moving.

Blading the Body - Strategically positioning your body at a 45-degree angle.

BOB - (See body opponent bag.)

Body Mechanics - Technically precise body movement during the execution of a body weapon, defensive technique, or other fighting maneuver.

Body Opponent Bag - (also known as BOB). A self standing, body-shaped punching bag constructed of synthetic rubber material called plastisol. The body opponent bag is comprised of two separate parts: the torso and base.

Body Weapon - (also known as tool). One of the various body parts that can be used to strike or otherwise injure or kill a criminal assailant.

Burn Out – A negative emotional state acquired by physically over training. Some symptoms include: illness, boredom, anxiety, disinterest in training, and general sluggishness.

C

Cadence - Coordinating tempo and rhythm to establish a timing pattern of movement.

Cardiorespiratory Conditioning - The component of physical fitness that deals with the heart, lungs, and circulatory system.

Centerline - An imaginary vertical line that divides your body in half and which contains many of your vital anatomical targets.

Circular Movement - Movements that follow the direction of a curve.

Clinching - Strategically locking up with the adversary while you are standing.

Close Quarter Combat - One of the three ranges of knife and bludgeon combat. At this distance, you can strike, slash, or stab your assailant with a variety of close-quarter techniques.

Cognitive Development - One of the five elements of CFA's mental component. The process of developing and enhancing your fighting skills through specific mental exercises and techniques. (See analysis and integration, killer instinct, philosophy and strategic/tactical development.)

Combat Oriented Training – Training that is specifically related to the harsh realities of both armed and unarmed combat. (see ritual oriented training and sport oriented training.)

Combative Arts - The various arts of war. (See martial arts.)

Combative Attributes - (See attributes of combat.)

Combative Fitness - A state characterized by cardiorespiratory and muscular/skeletal conditioning, as well as proper body composition.

Combat Ranges - The various ranges of unarmed combat.

Combative Utility - The quality of condition of being combatively useful.

Combination(s) - (See compound attack.)

Compound Attack - One of the five conventional methods of attack. Two or more body weapons launched in strategic succession whereby the fighter overwhelms his assailant with a flurry of full speed, full force blows.

Conditioning Training - A CFA training methodology requiring the practitioner to deliver a variety of offensive and defensive combinations for a four minute period (See proficiency training and street training.)

Contemporary Fighting Arts® (CFA) - A modern martial art and self-defense system made up of three parts: physical, mental, and spiritual.

Coordination - A physical attribute characterized by the ability to perform a technique or movement with efficiency, balance, and accuracy.

Counterattack - Offensive action made to counter an assailant's initial attack.

Cross Stepping - The process of crossing one foot in front or behind the other when moving.

D

Defense - The ability to strategically thwart an assailant's attack (armed or unarmed).

Diet - A life-style of healthy eating.

Distancing - The ability to quickly understand spatial relationships and how they relate to combat.

Double-End Bag – A small leather ball suspended in the air by bungee cord which develops striking accuracy, speed, timing, eye-hand coordination, footwork and overall defensive skills.

E

Effectiveness - One of the three criteria for a CFA body weapon, technique, tactic or maneuver. It means the ability to produce a desired effect (See efficiency and safety.)

Efficiency - One of the three criteria for a CFA body weapon, technique, tactic or maneuver. It means the ability to reach an objective quickly and economically (see effectiveness and safety.)

Evasion - A defensive maneuver that allows you to strategically maneuver your body away from the assailant's strike.

Evasive Sidestepping - Evasive footwork where the practitioner moves to either the right or left side.

Evasiveness - A combative attribute. The ability of avoid threat or danger.

Excessive Force - An amount of force that exceeds the need for a particular event and is unjustified in the eyes of the law.

Experimentation - The painstaking process of testing a combative hypothesis or theory.

Explosiveness - A combative attribute that is characterized by a sudden outburst of violent energy.

F

Fighting Stance - One of the different types of stances used in CFA's system. A strategic posture you can assume when face-to-face with an unarmed assailant (s). The fighting stance is generally used after you have launched your first strike tool.

Finesse - A combative attribute. The ability to skillfully execute a movement or a series of movements with grace and refinement.

Fisted blows – Hand blows delivered with a clenched fist.

Fist loading - The process of delivering fisted blows with kubotan in your hand.

Flexibility - The muscles' ability to move through maximum natural ranges (See muscular/skeletal conditioning.)

Focus Mitts – Durable leather hands mitts used to develop and sharpen offensive and defensive skills.

Footwork - Quick, economical steps performed on the balls of the feet while you are relaxed, alert, and balanced. Footwork is structured around four general movements: forward, backward, right, and left.

G

Grappling Range - One of the three ranges of unarmed combat. Grappling range is the closest distance of unarmed combat from which you can employ a wide variety of close-quarter tools and techniques. The grappling range of unarmed combat is also divided into two different planes: vertical (standing) and horizontal (ground fighting). (See kicking range and punching range.)

Grappling Range Tools - The various body tools and techniques that are employed in the grappling range of unarmed combat, including head butts; biting, tearing, clawing, crushing, and gouging tactics; foot stomps, horizontal, vertical, and diagonal elbow strikes, vertical and diagonal knee strikes, chokes, strangles, joint locks, and holds. (See punching range tools and kicking range tools.)

H

Hand Positioning - (See guard.)

Hand Wraps – Long strips of cotton that are wrapped around the hands and wrists for greater protection.

Head-Hunter - A fighter who primarily attacks the head.

Heavy Bag - A large cylindrical shaped bag that is used to develop kicking, punching or striking power.

High-Line Kick - One of the two different classifications of a kick. A kick that is directed to targets above an assailant's waist level. (See low-line kick.)

Hook Kick - A circular kick that can be delivered in both kicking and punching ranges.

Hook Punch - A circular punch that can be delivered in both the punching and grappling ranges.

I

Impact Power - Destructive force generated by mass and velocity.

Incapacitate - To disable an assailant by rendering him unconscious or damaging his bones, joints or organs.

J

Jiu-jitsu – Translates to "soft/pliable". Jiu-jitsu is a martial art developed in feudal Japan that emphasizes throws, joint locks and weapons training.

Joint Lock - A grappling range technique that immobilizes the assailant's joint.

Judo - Translates to "gentle/soft way". Judo is an Olympic sport which originated in Japan.

K

Kick - A sudden, forceful strike with the foot.

Kicking Range - One of the three ranges of unarmed combat. Kicking range is the furthest distance of unarmed combat wherein you use your legs to strike an assailant. (See grappling range and punching range.)

Kicking Range Tools - The various body weapons employed in the kicking range of unarmed combat, including side kicks, push kicks, hook kicks, and vertical kicks.

Kubotan - A close-quarter self-defense weapon.

L

Lead Side -The side of the body that faces an assailant.

Linear Movement - Movements that follow the path of a straight line.

Low Maintenance Tool - Offensive and defensive tools that require the least amount of training and practice to maintain proficiency. Low maintenance tools generally do not require preliminary stretching.

Low-Line Kick - One of the two different classifications of a kick. A kick that is directed to targets below the assailant's waist level. (See high-line kick.)

Lock - (See joint lock.)

M

Maneuver - To manipulate into a strategically desired position.

Martial arts - The "arts of war".

Self-Defense Tips and Tricks

Mechanics - (See body mechanics.)

Mental Attributes - The various cognitive qualities that enhance your fighting skills.

Mental Component - One of the three vital components of the CFA system. The mental component includes the cerebral aspects of fighting including the Killer Instinct, Strategic & Tactical Development, Analysis & Integration, Philosophy and Cognitive Development (See physical component and spiritual component.)

Mixed Martial Arts - Also known as MMA, is a concept of fighting where the practitioner integrates a variety of fighting styles into a single method of fighting that can be tested in a regulated full-contact combat sport.

Mobility - A combative attribute. The ability to move your body quickly and freely while balanced. (See footwork.)

Modern Martial Art - A pragmatic combat art that has evolved to meet the demands and characteristics of the present time.

Muscular Endurance - The muscles' ability to perform the same motion or task repeatedly for a prolonged period of time.

Muscular Flexibility - The muscles' ability to move through maximum natural ranges.

Muscular Strength - The maximum force that can be exerted by a particular muscle or muscle group against resistance.

Muscular/Skeletal Conditioning - An element of physical fitness that entails muscular strength, endurance, and flexibility.

N

Neutral Zone - The distance outside of the kicking range from which neither the practitioner nor the assailant can touch the other.

No Holds Barred Competition (NHB) – A sport competition with few rules.

Non telegraphic Movement - Body mechanics or movements that do not inform an assailant of your intentions.

O

Offense - The armed and unarmed means and methods of attacking a criminal assailant.

Offensive Flow - Continuous offensive movements (kicks, blows, and strikes) with unbroken continuity that ultimately neutralize or terminate the opponent. (See compound attack.)

Offensive Reaction Time (ORT) - The elapsed time between target selection and target impaction.

P

Pain Tolerance - Your ability to physically and psychologically withstand pain.

Parry - A defensive technique; a quick, forceful slap that redirects an assailant's linear attack. There are two types of parries: horizontal and vertical.

Patience - A combative attribute. The ability to endure and tolerate difficulty.

Perception - Interpretation of vital information acquired from your senses when faced with a potentially threatening situation.

Physical Attributes - The numerous physical qualities that enhance your combative skills and abilities.

Physical Component - One of the three vital components of the CFA system. The physical component includes the physical aspects of fighting including Physical Fitness, Weapon/Technique Mastery, and Combative Attributes. (See mental component and spiritual component.)

Physical Conditioning - (See combative fitness.)

Physical Fitness - (See combative fitness.)

Positioning - The spatial relationship of the assailant to the assailed person in terms of target exposure, escape, angle of attack, and various other strategic considerations.

Power - A physical attribute of armed and unarmed combat. The amount of force you can generate when striking an anatomical target.

Power Generators – Specific points on your body which generate impact power. There are three anatomical power generators: shoulders, hips, and feet.

Precision - (See accuracy.)

Preparedness – A state of being ready for combat. There are

three components of preparedness: affective preparedness, cognitive preparedness and psychomotor preparedness.

Proficiency Training - A CFA training methodology requiring the practitioner to execute a specific body weapon, technique, maneuver or tactic over and over for a prescribed number or repetitions. (See conditioning training and street training.)

Proxemics - The study of the nature and effect of man's personal space.

Proximity - The ability to maintain a strategically safe distance from a threatening individual.

Psychological Conditioning - The process of conditioning the mind for the horrors and rigors of real combat.

Punch - A quick, forceful strike of the fists.

Punching Range - One of the three ranges of unarmed combat. Punching range is the mid range of unarmed combat from which the fighter uses his hands to strike his assailant. (See kicking range and grappling range.)

Punching Range Tools - The various body weapons that are employed in the punching range of unarmed combat, including finger jabs, palm heel strikes, rear cross, knife hand strikes, horizontal and shovel hooks, uppercuts, and hammer fist strikes. (See grappling range tools and kicking range tools.)

Q

Qualities of Combat - (See attributes of combat.)

R

Range - The spatial relationship between a fighter and a threatening assailant.

Range Deficiency - The inability to effectively fight and defend in all ranges (armed and unarmed) of combat.

Range Manipulation - A combative attribute. The strategic manipulation of combat ranges.

Range Proficiency - A combative attribute. The ability to effectively fight and defend in all ranges (armed and unarmed) of combat.

Ranges of Engagement - (See combat ranges.)

Ranges of Unarmed Combat - The three distances a fighter might physically engage with an assailant while involved in unarmed combat: kicking range, punching range, and grappling range.

Raze – To level, demolish or obliterate.

Razer – One who performs the Razing methodology.

Razing – The second phase of the WidowMaker Program. A series of vicious close quarter techniques designed to physically and psychologically extirpate a criminal attacker.

Reaction Dynamics - The assailant's physical response or reaction to a particular tool, technique, or weapon after initial contact is made.

Reaction Time - The elapsed time between a stimulus and the response to that particular stimulus (See offensive reaction time and defensive reaction time.)

Rear Cross - A straight punch delivered from the rear hand that crosses from right to left (if in a left stance) or left to right (if in a right stance).

Rear Side - The side of the body furthest from the assailant (See lead side.)

Refinement - The strategic and methodical process of improving or perfecting.

Repetition - Performing a single movement, exercise, strike or action continuously for a specific period.

Rhythm - Movements characterized by the natural ebb and flow of related elements.

S

Safety - One of the three criteria for a CFA body weapon, technique, maneuver or tactic. It means the that the tool, technique, maneuver or tactic provides the least amount of danger and risk for the practitioner (See efficiency and effectiveness.)

Self-Confidence - Having trust and faith in yourself.

Set - A term used to describe a grouping of repetitions.

Shadow Fighting - A CFA training exercise used to develop and refine your tools, techniques, and attributes of armed and unarmed combat.

Skeletal Alignment - The proper alignment or arrangement of your body. Skeletal Alignment maximizes the structural integrity of striking tools.

Skills – One of the three factors that determine who will win a street fight. Skills refers to psychomotor proficiency with the tools and techniques of combat. (See Attitude and Knowledge.)

Slipping - A defensive maneuver that permits you to avoid an assailant's linear blow without stepping out of range. Slipping can be accomplished by quickly snapping the head and upper torso sideways (right or left) to avoid the blow.

Snap Back - A defensive maneuver that permits you to avoid an assailant's linear and circular blow without stepping out of range. The snap back can be accomplished by quickly snapping the head backwards to avoid the assailant's blow.

Sparring – A training exercise where two (or more) fighters fight each other while wearing protective equipment.

Speed - A physical attribute of armed and unarmed combat. The rate or a measure of the rapid rate of motion.

Spiritual Component - One of the three vital components of the CFA system. The spiritual component includes the metaphysical issues and aspects of existence (See physical component and mental component.)

Sport Oriented Training – Training that is geared for competition that is governed by a set of rules. (See combat oriented training and ritual oriented training.)

Sprawling – A grappling technique used to counter a double or single leg takedown.

Square-Off - To be face-to-face with the body opponent bag.

Stance - One of the many strategic postures that you assume prior to or during armed or unarmed combat.

Strategic/Tactical development - One of the five elements of CFA's mental component.

Strategy - A carefully planned method of achieving your goal of engaging an assailant under advantageous conditions.

Street Fight - A spontaneous and violent confrontation between two or more individuals wherein no rules apply.

Street Fighter - An unorthodox combatant who has no formal training. His combative skills and tactics are usually developed in the street by the process of trial and error.

Street Training - A CFA training methodology requiring the practitioner to deliver explosive compound attacks for ten to twenty-seconds (See conditioning training and proficiency training.)

Strength Training - The process of developing muscular strength through systematic application of progressive resistance.

Striking Art - A combat art that relies predominantly on striking techniques to neutralize or terminate a criminal attacker.

Striking Tool - A natural body weapon that impacts with the assailant's anatomical target.

Strong Side - The strongest and most coordinated side of your body.

Structure - A definite and organized pattern.

Style - The distinct manner in which a fighter executes or performs his combat skills.

Stylistic Integration - The purposeful and scientific collection of tools and techniques from various disciplines, which are strategically integrated and dramatically altered to meet three essential criteria: efficiency, effectiveness, and combative safety.

Submission Hold – (also known as control and restraint techniques). Many of the locks and holds that create sufficient pain to cause the adversary to submit.

Submission Technique - Includes all locks, bars, and holds that cause sufficient pain to cause the adversary to submit.

System - The unification of principles, philosophies, rules, strategies, methodologies, tools, and techniques or a particular method of combat.

T

Tactic - The skill of using the available means to achieve an end.

Target Awareness - A combative attribute which encompasses 5 strategic principles: target orientation, target recognition, target selection, target impaction, and target exploitation.

Target Exploitation - A combative attribute. The strategic maximization of your assailant's reaction dynamics during a fight. Target Exploitation can be applied in both armed and unarmed encounters.

Target Impaction - The successful striking of the appropriate anatomical target.

Target Orientation - A combative attribute. Having a workable knowledge of the assailant's anatomical targets.

Target Recognition - The ability to immediately recognize appropriate anatomical targets during an emergency self-defense situation.

Target Selection - The process of mentally selecting the appropriate anatomical target for your self-defense situation. This is predicated on certain factors, including proper force response, assailant's positioning and range.

Technique - A systematic procedure by which a task is accomplished.

Telegraphing - Unintentionally making your intentions known to your adversary.

Tempo - The speed or rate at which you speak.

Timing - A physical and mental attribute or armed and unarmed combat. Your ability to execute a movement at the optimum moment.

Tool - (See body weapon.)

Traditional Martial Arts - Any martial art that fails to evolve and change to meet the demands and characteristics of its present environment.

Traditional Style/System - (See traditional martial art.)

Training Drills - The various exercises and drills aimed at perfecting combat skills, attributes, and tactics.

U

Unified Mind - A mind free and clear of distractions and focused on the combative situation.

Use of Force Response - A combative attribute. Selecting the appropriate level of force for a particular emergency self-defense situation.

V

Visualization – Also known as Mental Visualization or Mental Imagery. The purposeful formation of mental images and scenarios in the mind's eye.

W

Warm-up - A series of mild exercises, stretches, and movement designed to prepare you for more intense exercise.

Weak Side - The weakest and most uncoordinated side of your body.

Weapon and Technique Mastery - A component of CFA's physical component. The kinesthetic and psychomotor development of a weapon or combative technique.

Webbing - A reinforced palm heel strike primarily delivered to the assailant's chin. It is termed Webbing because your hands resemble a large web that wraps around the enemy's face.

WidowMaker Program – A fighting style created by Sammy Franco that is specifically designed to teach the law-abiding citizen how to use extreme force when faced with immediate threat of unlawful deadly criminal attack. The WidowMaker program is divided into two sections or phases: Webbing and Razing.

Y

Yell - A loud and aggressive scream or shout used for various strategic reasons.

Z

Zero Beat – One of the four beat classifications of the Widow-Maker Program. Zero beat strikes are full pressure techniques applied to a specific target until it completely ruptures. Zero beat tools include gouging, biting and choking techniques

Zone One - Anatomical targets related to your senses, including the eyes, temple, nose, chin, and back of neck.

Zone Two - Anatomical targets related to your breathing, including front of neck, solar plexus, ribs, and groin.

Zone Three - Anatomical targets related to your mobility, including thighs, knees, shins, and instep.

About The Author

With over 30 years of experience, Sammy Franco is one of the world's foremost authorities on armed and unarmed self-defense. Highly regarded as a leading innovator in combat sciences, Mr. Franco was one of the premier pioneers in the field of "reality-based" self-defense and martial arts instruction.

Sammy Franco is perhaps best known as the founder and creator of Contemporary Fighting Arts (CFA), a state-of-the-art offensive-based combat system that is specifically designed for real-world self-defense. CFA is a sophisticated and practical system of self-defense, designed specifically to provide efficient and effective methods to avoid, defuse, confront, and neutralize both armed and unarmed attackers.

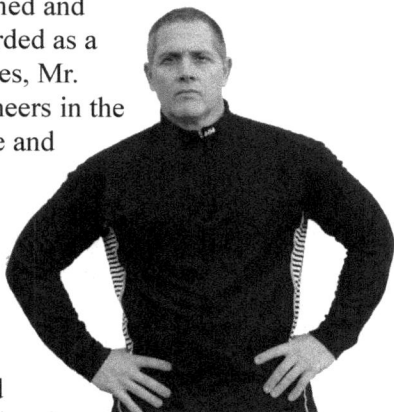

CFA also draws from the concepts and principles of numerous sciences and disciplines, including police and military science, criminal justice, criminology, sociology, human psychology, philosophy, histrionics, kinesics, proxemics, kinesiology, emergency medicine, crisis management, and human anatomy.

Sammy Franco has frequently been featured in martial art magazines, newspapers, and appeared on numerous radio and television programs. Mr. Franco has also authored numerous books, magazine articles and editorials, and has developed a popular library of instructional videos.

Sammy Franco's experience and credibility in the combat science is unequaled. One of his many accomplishments in this field includes the fact that he has earned the ranking of a Law Enforcement Master Instructor, and has designed, implemented, and taught officer survival training to the United States Border Patrol (USBP). He instructs members of the US Secret Service, Military Special Forces,

Washington DC Police Department, Montgomery County, Maryland Deputy Sheriffs, and the US Library of Congress Police. Sammy Franco is also a member of the prestigious International Law Enforcement Educators and Trainers Association (ILEETA) as well as the American Society of Law Enforcement Trainers (ASLET) and he is listed in the "Who's Who Director of Law Enforcement Instructors."

Sammy Franco is a nationally certified Law Enforcement Instructor in the following curricula: PR-24 Side-Handle Baton, Police Arrest and Control Procedures, Police Personal Weapons Tactics, Police Power Handcuffing Methods, Police Oleoresin Capsicum Aerosol Training (OCAT), Police Weapon Retention and Disarming Methods, Police Edged Weapon Countermeasures and "Use of Force" Assessment and Response Methods.

Mr. Franco is also a National Rifle Association (NRA) instructor who specializes in firearm safety, personal protection and advanced combat pistol shooting.

Mr. Franco holds a Bachelor of Arts degree in Criminal Justice from the University of Maryland. He is a regularly featured speaker at a number of professional conferences, and conducts dynamic and enlightening seminars on numerous aspects of self-defense and personal protection.

For more information about Mr. Franco and his unique Contemporary Fighting Arts system, you can visit his website at: www.SammyFranco.com

If you liked this book, you will also want to read these:

WHEN SECONDS COUNT
Self-Defense for the Real World
by Sammy Franco

When Seconds Count is a comprehensive street smart self-defense book instructing law abiding citizens how to protect themselves against the mounting threat of violent crime. When Seconds Count is considered by many to be one of the best books on real world self-defense instruction. Ideal for men and women of all ages who are serious about taking responsibility for their own safety. By studying the concepts and techniques taught in this book, you will feel a renewed sense of empowerment, enabling you to live your life with greater confidence and personal freedom. 10 x 7, paperback, photos, illustrations, 208 pages.

KUBOTAN POWER
Quick and Simple Steps to Mastering the Kubotan Keychain
by Sammy Franco

In this unique book, world-renowned self-defense expert, Sammy Franco takes thirty years of real-world teaching experience and gives you quick, easy and practical kubotan techniques that can be used by civilians, law enforcement personnel, or military professionals. Kubotan Power teaches you: tactical flashlight conversions, combat applications, grips, essential do's and don'ts, weapon nomenclature, impact shock, self-defense stages, high and low concealment positions, weapon deployment, target awareness, vital targets and medical implications, use of force considerations, attributes of fighting, defensive techniques, takedowns, training and flow drills, ground fighting, and much more. Whether you are a beginner or advanced, student or instructor, Kubotan Power shows you how to protect yourself and your loved ones against any thug you're likely to encounter on the street. 8.5 x 5.5, paperback, photos, illustrations, 204 pages.

THE COMPLETE BODY OPPONENT BAG BOOK
by Sammy Franco

In this one-of-a-kind book, world-renowned martial arts expert, Sammy Franco teaches you the many hidden training features of the body opponent bag that will improve your fighting skills and accelerate your fitness and conditioning. Develop explosive speed and power, improve your endurance, and tone, and strengthen your entire body. With detailed photographs, step-by-step instructions, and dozens of unique workout routines, The Complete Body Opponent Bag Book is the authoritative resource for mastering this lifelike punching bag. 8.5 x 5.5, paperback, photos, illustrations, 206 pages.

FIRST STRIKE
End a Fight in Ten Seconds or Less!
by Sammy Franco

Learn how to stop any attack before it starts by mastering the art of the preemptive strike. First Strike gives you an easy-to-learn yet highly effective self-defense game plan for handling violent close-quarter combat encounters. First Strike will teach you instinctive, practical and realistic self-defense techniques that will drop any criminal attacker to the floor with one punishing blow. By reading this book and by practicing, you will learn the hard-hitting skills necessary to execute a punishing first strike and ultimately prevail in a self-defense situation. And that's what it is all about: winning in as little time as possible. 8.5 x 5.5, paperback, photos, illustrations, 202 pages.

WAR MACHINE
How to Transform Yourself Into A Vicious & Deadly Street Fighter
by Sammy Franco

War Machine is a book that will change you for the rest of your life! When followed accordingly, War Machine will forge your mind, body and spirit into iron. Once armed with the mental and physical attributes of the War Machine, you will become a strong and confident warrior that can handle just about anything that life may throw your way. In essence, War Machine is a way of life. Powerful, intense, and hard. 11 x 8.5, paperback, photos, illustrations, 210 pages.

OUT OF THE CAGE
A Complete Guide to Beating a Mixed Martial Artist on the Street
by Sammy Franco

Forget the UFC! The truth is, a street fight is the "ultimate no holds barred fight" often with deadly consequences, but you don't need to join a mixed martial arts school or become a cage fighter to defeat a mixed martial artist on the street. What you need are solid skills and combat proven techniques that can be applied under the stress of real world combat conditions. Out of the Cage takes you inside the mind of the MMA fighter and reveals all of his weaknesses, allowing you to quickly exploit them to your advantage. 10 x 7, paperback, photos, illustrations, 194 pages.

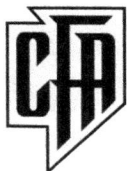

www.ingramcontent.com/pod-product-compliance
Lightning Source LLC
Chambersburg PA
CBHW072013290326
41934CB00007BA/1131